The International Lil

BIOLOGICAL MEMORY

Founded by C. K. Ogden

The International Library of Psychology

COGNITIVE PSYCHOLOGY
In 21 Volumes

BIOLOGICAL MEMORY

EUGENIO RIGNANO

Introduction by E W MacBride

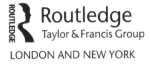

Routledge
Taylor & Francis Group

LONDON AND NEW YORK

First published in 1926 by
Routledge, Trench, Trubner & Co., Ltd.
2 Park Square, Milton Park, Abingdon, Oxfordshire OX14 4RN
711 Third Avenue, New York, NY 10017

First issued in paperback 2014

Routledge is an imprint of the Taylor and Francis Group, an informa business

British Library Cataloguing in Publication Data
A CIP catalogue record for this book
is available from the British Library

Biological Memory
ISBN 0415-20971-4
Cognitive Psychology: 21 Volumes
ISBN 0415-21126-3
The International Library of Psychology: 204 Volumes
ISBN 0415-19132-7

ISBN 13: 978-1-138-87504-3 (pbk)
ISBN 13: 978-0-415-20971-7 (hbk)

CONTENTS

CONTENTS

INTRODUCTION

to the English Translation

by

Professor E. W. MacBride, D.Sc., F.R.S.

In offering to English readers a translation of Prof. Rignano's work, "Biological Memory," we should like to call attention to two facts—first, that the title conveys no adequate idea of the importance of the theory set forth in it ; Prof. Rignano aims at nothing less than an exhaustive analysis of the differences which distinguish living from non-living substance and he attempts to account for these differences as the manifold effects of a single quality ; and secondly, he acknowledges in the preface that although he has dealt with all the phenomena of life including those of mind, he is not a specialist in these matters, but has considered them from the philosophic point of view.

If we consider the second point first, we may support Prof. Rignano's plea that in treating of such fundamental questions as the nature of life, there is room for the synthetic philosopher who is able to take a broad outlook over the whole field and to emphasise what appear to him to be the real points at issue. In the present state of science, when such extreme specialisation is necessary in order to make it possible for the researcher to obtain any results at all within the span of a human life, the outlook of the scientific worker is apt to be so restricted that he is unable to see the wood for the trees. But the synthetic philosopher labours under the great disadvantage of having to take all his facts second-hand ; and consequently is liable to base his conclusions on observations which workers in the subject consider obsolete or badly attested. Prof. Rignano is acutely conscious of this handicap and he expressly puts forward his theory as a provisional hypothesis, which he expects to be subjected to much criticism ; nay more he invites criticism by the experts in special fields in order that he may be in a position to modify his views so as to bring them into better accordance with ascertained facts.

If Prof. Rignano really had been able to elaborate a theory of life which was complete and satisfactory in all its details, he would have succeeded in solving one of the main problems of our existence ; and such fortune is greater than Nature allots to any man. To none of us is granted more than to lift a small corner of the covering concealing that veiled Isis the Truth ; whilst those of us who have succeeded in doing so are too apt to imagine that what we have thus revealed is the whole truth instead of only a small part of it. It is instructive to observe how every discoverer of a new principle strives to apply it to the solution of every possible question, in a word, to run it to death. In his enthusiasm for the new truth, its first promulgater inevitably damages it ; for his opponents fasten on the cases to which he tries to apply it where it does not apply and thus they attempt to bring the whole thing into discredit.

We now revert to the first point which we emphasised viz., the theory itself, and we may say at once that although we consider that this will require much modification in detail, we regard it as an astoundingly successful effort to analyse vital phenomena. If it is not the truth, it at least bears a strong resemblance to what the truth must be. It may be divided into two parts, the biological and the psychological; in what follows we shall deal almost exclusively with the biological portion; leaving to other experts the task of criticising the psychological part. We cannot refrain, however, from remarking that we consider Prof. Rignano's analysis of mental functions extraordinarily interesting and suggestive; his methods of interpreting reason, attention and will are in many ways clearer and more convincing than any which we have so far encountered in the writings of other psychologists. But we must register our entire dissent from his scornful dismissal of metaphysical reasoning. If this translation is as widely read as we hope it will be, we anticipate that Prof. Rignano's remarks will provoke such a " repercussion " on the part of metaphysicians as will induce him to modify his position. Metaphysics which deals with the subjective element in experience has as good a justification for itself as science which deals with the objective factor.

If we now examine the biological portion of Prof. Rignano's theory we find that he discovers the essential difference between living and non-living things to be this :—living things remember, dead matter does not remember. But the word " memory " is employed by us to denote two different things. When we recall past experiences—faces that we have seen and places that we have visited in the past—we are said to remember them, and this may be termed sensorial memory. When again we have learnt to play a game like tennis, or acquired an accomplishment such as swimming, in our youth, and for many years have had no opportunity of exercising our skill in either respect, then if in middle life we are called on either to play tennis or to swim we shall find that a great deal of the skill which we once acquired, though not all, still remains with us ; this may be termed habitudinal memory. We as living beings possess both kinds of memory, but when memory is regarded as a universal attribute of living substance, it is of course habitudinal memory that is meant. So far as we yet know we are not justified in attributing sensorial memory to an oak tree.

Prof. Rignano terms his theory "centro-epigenetic;" by this he means that the fertilised egg embodies in its nucleus all the memories acquired during the past history of the race, and that when it begins to develop, all these memories are handed on to the daughter nuclei which are developed from the division of the egg-nucleus intact, but that very soon one part of the growing embryo acquires a dominance over the rest and so to speak leads in the development. This governance Prof. Rignano pictures as a series of impulses emitted by the nuclei of the central zone which radiate out to all parts of the organism and control its development ; the nuclei outside this zone are supposed to have their powers gradually suppressed and to be eventually reduced to a specialised condition in which they no longer possess more than a fraction of their original potencies.

The paths along which these influences radiate are supposed to be the intercellular bridges connecting cells together. As the animal grows and increases in complication of structure, some of these bridges are converted into nervous fibres, and in animals which have a developed nervous system the central zone is supposed to be constituted by a portion of this system. The trophic influence of the nervous system in animals which possess it is supposed to prove that all influences by means of which one part governs the development of another are at bottom of a nervous nature.

When an organism encounters a new condition of the environment it is not passively changed as a similar piece of dead substance would be, but it "reacts," that is, it responds to the change by an active output of energy. This is termed a "reaction." Now Rignano assumes that a reaction leaves some kind of trace of itself in all the nuclei of the body including those of the central zone. This trace is what is termed memory. It has the power of facilitating the reproduction of the reaction which called it forth—so that this reaction occurs the second time as a response to a slighter stimulus or is even evoked by a portion only of the stimulus which originally called it into being. This recurrence of a reaction as a result of the return of a portion of the original condition is termed "ecphory," a name invented by Semon.

The germ cells do not form part of the central zone

of the animal, but they receive materials emitted by the nuclei of the cells constituting this zone. These latter contain the real effective germinal substance ; that is the substance made up of the various specific mnemonic accumulations which constitute phylogenetic memory. When the germ cells develop, the " traces " which they contain become active one after another, and bring about responses in the growth of the embryo which cause it to pass through a series of stages which represent the stages through which the race passed when these memories were originally acquired.

" Instincts " are but the engrained memories of former " voluntary " reactions ; when the memory-traces become very powerful owing to the accumulation produced by an enormous number of repetitions carried out through numberless generations, then they are able to produce the appropriate reaction in response to a very slight stimulus or in the absence of a stimulus. Thus is explained the existence of instincts designed for future purposes of which the animal in which they become active can have no knowledge, as when, for instance, the Ichneumon fly pierces the body of the caterpillar in order to lay its egg which will develop into the fly which the mother will never see.

Now the main outlines of Rignano's views have been experimentally proved to be correct. That habits called forth as reactions to a changed environment become easier with constant repetition, we all know as a result of our own experience, but few realise that in the last twenty years the fact that the results of habit are carried over into the offspring has been experimentally demonstrated by carefully devised

6

crucial experiments. The possibility of this transmission was dogmatically denied by Weismann, on the ground of his own crude theoretical conceptions of the structure of protoplasm—a conception which has been made to look ludicrous by the researches of Hertwig, Driesch and others of that school ; and this dogma uncritically copied from text-book to text-book has acquired in many zoological minds something of the fixity of a religious tradition ; it has indeed awakened what Rignano would call a strong " affectivity " in its support and those imbued with this " affectivity " have left no stone unturned to damage the credit of the results which overturn their favourite dogma.

Kammerer in Vienna and Durkhen in Breslau have both shown that in animals which react to differences in illumination by a change in their skin colour, this reaction occurs in greatly increased degree if a second generation is exposed to the same conditions as their parents, and even when the second generation are returned to what may be called the typical conditions of the species, the reaction still shows itself *especially during the earlier stages of growth* though, of course, in lessened degree.

Durkhen worked with the pupæ of the white butterfly. These pupæ have usually an integument of a chalky white colour, but in about 4 per cent. the cuticle is transparent and then the animal appears green owing to its green blood shining through. When these pupæ are exposed during the process of pupation to orange light the formation of this chalky white pigment is interfered with and 65 per cent become green ; when a second generation are exposed to similar conditions, 95 per cent. become green ; and when this generation are reared in ordinary daylight, 34 per cent. still become green. Durkhen's results have been repeated on the peacock butterfly (*Vanessa io*) in Vienna by Miss Brecher and confirmed.

Kammerer worked with the spotted Salamander (*Salamandra maculosa*), which in two generations he converted into a form indistinguishable from the black Salamander (*S. atra*). In addition, he succeeded in a marvellous way in " ecphorising " lost habits in the midwife toad (*Alytes obstetricans*) and in the blind cave-newt (*Proteus anguineus*). The midwife toad in contradistinction to all other toads pairs on land, and the skin of the female remains dry and horny ; the male therefore experiences no difficulty in retaining a hold on his partner and he is devoid of the horny pad on his hand which other male toads which pair in water have developed in order to enable them to keep the slippery female within their embraces. But the midwife toad is without any doubt a secondary modification of the ordinary type of water-inhabiting toad, and Kammerer succeeded in accustoming the midwife toad to pair in water and in five generations he successfully " ecphorised " the horny pad in the male. The blind cave-newt has lost its eyes by a sojourn for thousands of years in complete darkness, but by subjecting the young to periods of illumination by ruby light Kammerer " ecphorised " perfect eyes endowed with powers of sight in one generation.

The Alytes with the horny pad and the Proteus with the large eyes were exhibited at the Linnean

8

INTRODUCTION

Society in London in 1923. Kammerer's critics in the vain attempt to discredit his evidence were driven to assert that in the ordinary amphibian the horny pad never appears on the palmar surface of the hand in amphibia, but only on the dorsal aspect! Surely a cause which is in need of such arguments is lost! Surely the distinguished biologist who made this statement had never demonstrated to an elementary class; it is impossible to look at a dozen frogs in the breeding season without seeing the extension of the pad to the palmar surface in most of them.

Herbert Spencer once termed the demonstration of the transmissibility or the non-transmissibility of the effects of habit, the cardinal problem in biology; for on its answer depends our estimate of the racial value of education, and of course the whole validity of Prof. Rignano's theory depends upon the assumption which Kammerer and Durkhen have shown to be correct.

The next point in Prof. Rignano's theory is that, in development, one particular portion of the embryo assumes the lead and dominates and controls the fate of the rest. Now this has also been proved to be literally true in many cases, and it is therefore a fair assumption that it is true in all. Spemann and his pupils have shown that in amphibian development the central zone is constituted by the dorsal lip of the blastopore in the gastrula stage. This dorsal lip in normal development forms a portion of the spinal cord. *Triton alpestris* and *Triton taeniatus* are two newts which produce eggs and embryos of different degrees of pigmentation. When a small portion of the dorsal lip of the blastopore of one species is grafted on to the upper part of the blastula of the second, it can be recognised by its pigmentation. The foreign tissue then controls the development of the egg with which it has been brought into contact and causes the formation of a spinal cord and notochord in the latter, starting from the position where the new tissue has been introduced.

The Ophiurid *Amphiura squamata* is a small brittle-star with a rounded disc and five arms radiating from the mouth, situated on the ventral surface. The disc contains the stomach and the genital organs. The whole disc is often spontaneously cast off, leaving only the framework of ossicles surrounding the mouth to which the arms are attached ; embedded in this framework is the highly developed nerve-ring. Starting from this basis the animal is able to re-generate a new disc, including the stomach, but the old disc cannot regenerate new arms.

The feather-star, *Antedon rosacea*, possesses a conical disc and ten graceful arms with lateral branches termed pinnules radiating out from the mouth. Surrounding the mouth is a slender nerve-ring comparable with the more highly developed nerve-ring of the brittle-star. In the apex of the disc however, opposite to the mouth, there is embedded an independent and much more powerful nervous system which is derived, not like the nerve-rings alluded to, from the skin, but from the wall of the body cavity. If the disc of the feather-star be gouged out and the whole of the alimentary canal, genital organs and nerve ring be removed, the activities of the animal are not much interfered with, and in a short time it regenerates an entirely new alimentary canal and nerve-ring, but if the large nerve centre situated in the apex is destroyed, the animal is permanently paralysed and soon dies. The main nervous system seems in all these cases to be the controlling factor in development.

The function of taste in mammals is carried out by minute " buds " of specialised sense-cells situated in the sides of the circumvallate papillæ of the tongue. These only appear in development when the branches of the seventh nerve reach the epidermis ; when these branches are cut the taste-buds speedily disappear.

The theory, however, that one part influences another in development by means of impulses of a nervous nature, emanating from the nuclei, requires a considerable amount of modification. First we must notice that one part of the embryo, besides acting on the rest by impulses of this kind, has also the power of influencing it by means of substances called " hormones " which are thrown into the circulation and carried to all parts of the body. Thus if the thyroid gland of a tadpole be cut out, the tadpole will grow in size, but will never metamorphose into a frog, but if such a tadpole is fed on the thyroid of an ox, metamorphosis speedily follows. If in a man the pituitary gland underneath the brain grows to an abnormal size, the man becomes a giant, whereas if it remain small the man remains a dwarf with infantile characteristics. It has been quite recently shown that this double method of transmitting influence exists in plants as well as in animals. In the sensitive plant irritation can be handed on when the living tissues are completely cut through and only the wood remains ; it is then carried by a chemical substance (hormone) dissolved in the water of the transpiration current. But a quicker influence is carried by the phloem which seem to act as a nervous system.

Secondly it is extremely doubtful if impulses can properly be said to proceed from the nucleus at all. An Amœba deprived of its nucleus continues to live for some time and exhibit all the characteristic reactions of the animal, but it is unable to assimilate food, repair waste and build up new protoplasm. It seems to be more just to regard it as the function of the nucleus to serve as a manufactory of new irritable substance by the explosion of which the impulses are produced.

Another view of Prof. Rignano's which requires modification is the theory that the nuclei lying outside the central zone become progressievly specialised as development goes on. Whilst it may be true that in old functional cells the nucleus may become specialised, it is then seen that the life of the cell in which it is contained is tending towards an end, for such nuclei cannot undergo regular division or rejuvenation. So long as a nucleus is capable of dividing by ordinary karyokinesis it shows by its definite and typical number of chromosomes that it has retained all the potencies of the original nucleus of the fertilized egg intact ; *what becomes specialised is not the nucleus but the cytoplasm.* In the development of the Ascidian Cynthia when the stage of the gastrula is reached there is along the dorsal lip of the blastopore a crescent of cells which Conklin calls chorda-neural cells because they give rise both to nerve cord and to notochord. Each cell has only a single nucleus, but each consists of two separate kinds of cytoplasm—a blueish and a clearer kind. At the next division of the cell the nucleus divides into two quite similar nuclei, but the clear protoplasm all goes into one daughter cell which is added to the growing nerve-cord, whilst the cell containing the blue protoplasm joins the developing notochord.

Thus the nucleus seems to preserve the powers of the whole organism in itself whether inside or outside the central zone, and the portion of these powers which will come to development seems to depend on local circumstances. This view which was put forward by Driesch, is accepted even by Morgan.

Prof. Rignano attempts to get nearer the nature of this faculty of memory exhibited by living organisms by attributing life itself to a special modification of energy, characterised by this property of leaving mnemonic traces behind it which distinguishes it from all other forms of energy. This special variety of energy is said to obey the general laws of energetics, that is to say, we presume, that it is convertible into other forms of energy.

This "vitalistico-energetic" hypothesis of Prof. Rignano will awaken, we doubt not, a great deal of interest and discussion. We do not think, however, that it can be upheld in its present form. We must ask at once what does Prof. Rignano mean by a "kind" of energy? Is not all energy at bottom one and the same, and are not its so-called modifications merely different manifestations caused by its association with aggregations of matter of different sizes ? When electrons move alone we have an electric current ; when they move in systems connected by protons, then we have atomic movement which is manifested by chemical reaction. When atoms move in connected aggregates then we have molecular movement or heat and finally when molecules move in connected masses we obtain the gross visible mechanical energy of motion. The *source* of the energy manifested in vital phenomena is to be found in the chemical energy of the food which the organism absorbs and in the energy of the medium in which it lives ; thus as we all know, the vital energy of green plants is derived from the radiant energy of sunlight and vital processes are nearly at a standstill in reptiles during the winter, but they wake up and become active with the returning heat of spring. After having operated in the living tissues the energy passes out again as mechanical movement, or is stored in potential form in the chemical energy of the products produced.

It would seem therefore to be more correct to say that energy manifests itself in a peculiar way when it enters living tissue, and the question arises what is the cause of this peculiarity. It seems to us that there are only two possible alternative answers to this question, and that there is no way of wedging a third alternative between them. Either the peculiarity is due to the way in which the atoms and molecules of the living substance are arranged in reference to one another, or there is in every organism a " something," an " entelechy " or " psychoid " which feels, remembers, and strives towards an end, which directs and combines forces, but is not itself a force. The first alternative is the materialistic or physico-chemical one, which was frankly adopted by Huxley, who defines an animal as a " molecular machine of great complexity " ; the second alternative is what Prof. Rignano calls the psycho-vitalistic one, which. though long under a cloud, has been revived and pressed with great force by Driesch and is adopted by our leading comparative psychologist, William MacDougall. Driesch shows in detail and Prof. Rignano would agree with him, that no machine could possibly be imagined which would perform like a living being ; and the only answer which his opponents can make is that whilst this is true now and here, yet in the future some supernal transcendental machine may be conceived of which will be adequate to the task !

On the other hand Driesch's " psychoid " or " entelechy " has been objected to as an empty word incapable of definition. Prof. Rignano enables us in some measure at least to answer this objection. We can say that an entelechy is a " group of memories." Further we can say that if, as every evolutionist believes, our own nature is akin to the nature of other living beings, then as no one, not even Sir Charles Sherrington himself, could or would deny that there is a " subject " in man, it is more natural to assume with MacDougall that there is some kind of a " subject " in the humblest amœba also, than to establish between man and his poorer relations an impassable chasm by confining the possession of mind to the human race.

Materialism as an explanation of human feelings

and actions proves to be so absurd when examined in detail that it cannot even be consistently stated. Even Huxley wavered, when he stated that " will " was non-material and that he was not a materialist because he could not conceive of the existence of matter without mind to picture it in.

It is of great interest that Prof. Rignano attempts to base an explanation of the affectivities and consequently of all the feelings which inspire and govern human action on biological memory, and we believe that he is in large measure right, for in the main we desire to retain what we are accustomed to, and " becoming accustomed " is habitudinal memory. Of course, this is not a complete explanation for it furnishes no account of the desire for novelty and change, but as we have already said we leave the detailed criticism of this part of Prof. Rignano's work to experts in psychology.

E. W. MacBride,

Imperial College of Science and Technology, London.

AUTHOR'S PREFACE

THE author of these essays is not a biologist in the ordinary sense of the word ; he has never worked in a laboratory, nor has he ever looked at a cell through the microscope, nor analysed chemically the product of a physiological process evoked by any kind of stimulus ; he has never made an experiment on muscular contraction or on the rapidity of transmission of nervous excitation. He is simply a " natural philosopher," who strives to unravel the theoretical significance of the results obtained by laboratory specialists, with the object of catching a glimpse of new analogies, of proceeding to new generalisations, of disclosing new horizons, of framing new hypotheses, in a word, of attempting to effect a synthesis and unification of the sciences of life.

If such is his function, and such are the contributions which he hopes to make to the progress of the sciences of life, the question at once arises : What are the advantages and what the disadvantages which he possesses as compared with the specialist in experimental science ? I shall endeavour to answer this question in the briefest manner, solely in order to justify myself for having ventured to give special thought to the most fundamental questions of life and consciousness, though I am not a specialist at all.

The reasons for considering the " theorist " or

" natural philosopher " inferior to the specialist in experimental science are certainly not negligible.

The former never possess the complete picture of the phenomena which constitute the subject-matter of his researches, since he only knows these through the information imparted to him by the experimenter. But what the latter describes and notes in his experiments and his observations constitute only a small part of what he has really seen and observed. A multitude of small details, of which the greater part have not been considered by the experimenter sufficiently important to be mentioned in his descriptions, and of which a large part have even almost escaped his notice, makes up, nevertheless, a precious background, which completes the picture of the development of the phenomenon. No verbal description, no drawing, and no photograph can ever reproduce in all its fullness the glittering spectacle which presents itself to the eager and admiring eyes of the observer. The theorist might be compared to a colour-blind man, who, in a landscape flooded with light, perceives only the dry and bald outlines of the things in it.

Besides, all these small details of secondary importance which the experimental specialist has observed, but which he has not described, all the unsuccessful experiments, all the proofs and controls which he has repeated before he has succeeded in finally establishing each of his results, and which have made up his own particular apprenticeship, all this precious material, of which nothing appears in the written account of his work, constitutes a rich harvest of facts of which the theorist necessarily remains for ever ignorant. The theorist, consequently, in each branch of science, is necessarily in possession of much less numerous details ; he is much less " master " of the subject ; much less confident in his statements about any given detail than the specialist.

The theorist, finally, cannot at once submit his own theories and hypotheses to the test of experiment, nor can he dissipate by means of direct observation the various doubts by which he is incessantly assailed. For each new experiment of which he has need, he must have recourse to the work of others, and for this work he must very often wait an indefinite time, and he finds it very difficult, even if he encounters the best of goodwill on the part of the experimenter, to arrange that this work shall be carried out along the lines and by the methods which he desires. Thus in very many cases the theorist is a little like the paralytic, who is unable to grasp or move anything that he sees before him, and therefore may remain for a long time uncertain as to the accuracy of his idea about any given object, which he only sees but cannot touch.

But if all these circumstances place the theorist in an inferior position to that occupied by the experimental specialist, there are other aspects of the case which make the position of the specialist inferior to that of the theorist.

For if we must admit that the more schematic and meagre pictures and representations which the theorist forms of phenomena, constitute from one point of view a disadvantage, seen from another standpoint they are real and peculiar advantages, in so far as they permit of a more generalised view of the phenomena in the place of the too concrete view which has become imprinted on the mind of the specialist as a result of his prolonged and careful observations.

Any schematic representation of facts is already a generalisation deduced from the observation of individual facts ; it is, in a word, a synthesis of the first order, and it constitutes the first and most important step toward the attainment of syntheses of higher orders.

The theorist, in his pursuit of ever wider generalisations and higher syntheses, has thus the advantage of beginning at a point more advanced than that reached by the specialist.

No longer encumbered with a multitude of individual facts and concrete details, which are actively present in the mind of the specialist, the theorist possesses a greater ease and facility of ascending still higher along the path of further generalisations and syntheses.

The theorist has also much wider opportunities of and much greater facility in getting into touch with the actual state of fundamental questions in quite different branches of science. His time is not taken up, even in minor degree, with actual manipulation ; in a single half-hour of reading he can become acquainted with results obtained by any particular specialist ; results, it may be, at which this specialist has only arrived after a full year of assiduous, long and difficult experimentation. Besides, when one considers the question of technique, so delicate, and at the same time so different in the various branches of science, and even in the different sub-divisions of the same branch, it must be admitted that the specialist finds great difficulty in passing from one order of phenomena to another. The long apprenticeship necessitated by the nature of certain researches, often leads the specialist to persist in following one line throughout his life, even if this is a very narrow one. On the other hand, if the power of getting into touch, by means of reading, with the essential features of any science requires for its attainment a real and specialised technique—though it may appear to the specialist to be much easier than it really is—it is at least the same for all classes of phenomena.

Consequently the theorist encounters no difficulty when he traverses all the divisions and sub-divisions of even a very wide field of research. It becomes thus easy to him to take in with a single glance even the most diverse sciences, and thus to bridge the wide abysses which still separate them.

The theorist, finally, is less exclusive, less one-sided, and more neutral in his point of view than the experimental specialist. The latter, in fact, does not proceed by chance in his observations and experiments, but is always guided, whether consciously or unconsciously, by some idea, conception or hypothesis, which is either his own, or which he has borrowed from someone else. Now, from the fact that he has been for a long time, during the whole period of his observations and experiments, an adherent of some dominant view, it results that this view becomes crystallised and changed into a mental habit sufficiently strong to overpower every other point of view which might conflict with it. The theorist, on the other hand, since he can take account of the most diverse and opposed points of view, and since he gives to the consideration of each in its turn the same time and the same amount of mental effort, does not polarise his mind in any particular direction, and does not feel himself irresistibly bound to one way of looking at things rather than another.

Thus he is better able to judge with serenity and impartiality the arguments and objections of each side, and so he often succeeds in extracting from the many points of view, all more or less one-sided, which he has examined, a less one-sided conception, which for that very reason will have more chance of corresponding better to what really exists.

Therefore, the theorist may often officiate as an impartial judge in the frequent, heated, and endless controversies in which different schools of specialists endeavour to gain decisive victory. He also sometimes succeeds in solving certain famous alleged antinomies, which are usually regarded as insoluble, but which, seen in the light of broader knowledge, turn out to be non-existent.

If the state of matters is really as we have described it, then we can understand that the tasks of the theorist and of the experimental specialist, instead of being mutually exclusive, are really complementary. The degree of dominant and capital importance which should and does characterise the work of the theorist in the biological and psychological sciences, even more than in the physical sciences, is due to the fact that in the former group of sciences the mass of individual facts to be systematised is much more complicated and confused than in the latter group. Further, in the former group, the independent sub-divisions of the subject are much more numerous and specialised ; and on that very account the need of co-ordination and synthesis is much more acute than in the latter group. This, indeed, is the point which we hope to prove, and to bring into greater prominence in the essays which we have collected in this volume.

Let us add that it is pre-eminently biology and psychology which more than any other sciences yield the highest degree of philosophic interest, because in a word, on them depend the solution of the questions of vitalism, of purpose in life, and of the relations between the soul and body. All of these are questions which, since Man has thought at all, have tormented philosophic minds. Moreover, since it is just these problems, with regard to which the specialist has nothing to say, which we have dared to consider in the pages which follow, we may hope that, even on this ground, the part which the theorist or " natural philosopher " has to play in biology and psychology in addition to, and with the object of synthesising the work of the specialists, will not be regarded as entirely useless.

E. R.

Milan, October, 1925.

BIOLOGICAL MEMORY

CHAPTER I

THE TRANSFORMIST HYPOTHESES LEAD TO THE MNEMONIC THEORIES OF DEVELOPMENT

Lamarck and Darwin. The individual variations on which natural selection works. The " particulate inheritance " of Galton. Preformed " gemmules." Weismann's theory of the continuity of germ-plasm. Weismann's deduction of the impossibility of the inheritance of acquired characters. Objections to the all-sufficiency of natural selection. The mutation theory of De Vries. The orthogenetic theories of Nägeli and Eimer. The steadily increasing number of observations and arguments in favour of the inheritability of acquired characters. The difficult question of the mechanism which effects this transmission. The recapitulation of phylogeny by ontogeny. The inevitable suggestion that this recapitulation is a mnemonic phenomenon. The first mnemonic ideas of Haeckel, Butler, Orr and Cope. The mnemonic theories of Hering and Semon. The necessity for the thorough investigation of the nature of " mnemonic " phenomena.

As everyone knows it was the French zoologist Lamarck who, at the beginning of the nineteenth century, first put forward a complete theory of the transformation of species. According to this theory it was the new efforts made by an organism to satisfy new needs which are due to the continual changes of the environment which produced corresponding morphological modifications in each species which underwent evolution.

Since these modifications are transmitted to posterity and, consequently, what every generation acquires becomes added to what the previous generation had acquired, it follows that each species should gradually become transformed into what would be regarded as another species. In this way one might conceive of all the living species being derived from the same ancestral stock.

But this theory of Lamarck which regarded the inheritability of acquired morphological modifications as the essential factor in the evolution of species, whilst it hardly mentioned natural selection at all except in some vague and unimportant statements, was for a long time practically ignored.

The famous book of Darwin on the Origin of Species which appeared about the middle of last century, was, on the contrary, as everyone knows, received with favour by the majority of naturalists and rapidly acquired wide-spread fame. Without denying the inheritability of the effects of use and disuse, Darwin pushed them into the background as factors in evolution in order to bring into prominence the factor of selection. Since that time, although Darwin had not mentioned Lamarck's name, Lamarck was rescued from oblivion and compared or, rather, contrasted with Darwin, because Lamarck had overlooked the factor of selection and had laid weight only on the other factor, viz., the inheritability of acquired modifications.

He benefited, even by this contrast, from all the fame which Darwin's theory had obtained ; so well, indeed, that there arose the two schools of the Neo-Lamarckians and the Neo-Darwinians who, as we know, still wage war with each other ; the former practically accepting only the factor of the inheritance of acquired characters, the latter admitting only the factor of selection.

It is easy to understand what a vast synthesis was constituted by the bare idea of the evolution of species, whatever factor in this evolutionary process one might consider the most important.

All living organisms were seen to belong to one enormous family. Man, that favourite of creation, stepped down from his high pedestal to mingle with the humble ranks of the animals.

The differences between animals and plants, that is to say between beings formerly considered animate and others which were considered inanimate, lost in its turn all appearance of substantial importance. No synthesis in the inorganic world had ever been broad enough to be compared with the synthesis effected by the transformist theory in the organic world.

Nevertheless, when the first stupefaction which was produced by the impact of so powerful a synthesis had passed away, people began to examine and analyse the contents of the new theory. Whilst this patient examination stimulated many to undertake new resarches in the most varied directions, in order to verify the more obvious postulates of and deductions from the theory, it at the same time gave rise to the creation of further subsidiary hypotheses in order to support the main theory. These hypotheses have attached very different branches of biological science to the main stem of the evolutionary theory, and have at the same time joined the various branches to each other.

Thus for instance since, according to Darwin, natural selection was supposed to act on purely fortuitous variations, which turned up not only amongst individuals of the same species or variety, but also amongst the offspring produced by the same pair of parents, it became necessary to concentrate attention on these variations. Galton's observations on the differences which distinguish the brothers of the same family from one another, led him to the discovery of the phenomenon which he named " particulate inheritance," a term which might be explained by the periphrasis, " the independent inheritability of different individual peculiarities."

This phenomenon appeared so striking that the necessity of attempting a further explanation of it became apparent. An explanation by the aid of hypothetical preformed germs was put forward ; that is to say, the hypothesis that, considering that each special characteristic could vary and be inherited independently of all the others, each must be represented in the seed or germ which corresponded to the whole organism by an infinitely small germ, distinct from the enormous number of other germs which corresponded to other characteristics. The " gemmules " of Darwin, the " pangenes " of De Vries and the " determinants " of Weismann are only so many different names which have been given to these hypothetical preformed germs. This preformist hypothesis of the germ led in turn to another hypothesis even more remarkable and fruitful, viz., that of Weismann on the continuity of the germ-plasm.

28

THE TRANSFORMIST HYPOTHESES

Darwin, indeed, had supposed that each cell of the organism, whether it had been produced in the ordinary way by the development of the individual, or whether it had been acquired after the development of the individual as a result of some new functional adaptation, produced its own gemmules and that these were carried about by the circulation of the blood, and were taken up by the genital organs, which he regarded simply as glands intended for the storing and re-emission of the germinal substance. But Galton transfused the blood of one variety of rabbit into the veins of another variety, and found that the descendant of the second variety never acquired the characters of the first, and he therefore concluded that this circulation of gemmules in the blood did not exist.

So he was led to consider that the germ-plasm was composed of an enormous number of different kinds of gemmules, that each kind of gemmule produced an indefinite number of others like itself which were incorporated in the germ-plasm, but that at the beginning of development only a very small proportion of gemmules, each of which could grow into a cell, took part in the formation of the body or " soma " ; the remainder, which Galton called the " stirp " (stock), was collected in a corner of the organism, in order to serve later as the " germ-plasm " of the organism.

It will be easily seen that this hypothesis is fundamentally the same as the famous theory of the " Continuity of the Germ-Plasm " of Weismann. Weismann in fact elaborated the theory of Galton and Darwin still further, and issued it in a more definite and perfect form.

We need not be astonished by the excitement, I had almost said the enthusiasm, with which Weismann's theory was received. So far as the development of organisms is concerned, the biologist finds himself confronted with two colossal difficulties, viz., (1) how the microscopic particle of matter which constitutes the germ-plasm can succeed in determining in its most minute details the structure of a complex organism such as a vertebrate, and (2) how such an organism in its turn can reproduce a small particle of matter endowed with the same astonishing properties.

Now the hypothesis of the continuity of the germ-plasm surmounted the second of these difficulties. According to this theory it was not the organism which formed anew the germ-plasm, but on the contrary it was the germ-plasm itself which, continually increased in quantity, maintained itself, and was transmitted from one organism to another without having undergone any qualitative alteration, and it was from the germ-plasm that small portions became successively detached in order to form one generation after another of the species. These generations consequently were not related to one another as mother to daughter, but were really only elder and younger sisters of each other.

But if the germ-plasm, after it had emitted the minute portion of itself destined to form the new organism, retired into a nook of the developing body and remained there unaltered until in due course it gave rise to the sexual cells of this body when the latter had become adult, then whatever modifications this body might undergo—modifications, that is to say, which had been acquired by the individual subsequent to birth as a consequence of some new functional adaptation—these modifications would not affect the germ-plasm   Such at least was the conclusion which has been drawn from the theory. Therefore acquired characters were not transmissible to subsequent generations.

Thus was born Neo-Darwinism or Weismannism ; a theory which denies, in the most uncompromising way, the kind of inheritance which the Lamarckian hypothesis makes into the mainspring of its working, and which Darwin himself accepted even though he attributed to it secondary importance.

However, old objections and still more formidable new ones were urged against the Weismannian doctrine that natural selection was the sole factor which had brought about evolution ; the polemics on this subject—of which the first and most brilliant, waged between Spencer and Weismann himself, l as become historic—eventually undermined the almost universal acceptance accorded to the theory of the non-transmissibility of acquired characters, which Weismann had enunciated and which the greater number of his followers regarded as implicitly involved in the doctrine of the continuity of the germ-plasm.

The difficulties which beset natural selection when it is put forward as the sole explanation of the marvellous structure of certain tissues and the shapes of certain organs and groups of organs strikingly adapted to their functions led to more careful study of the nature and manifestations of structural adaptation, and brought into prominence the importance of simultaneous and co-ordinated variations, which natural selection is incapable of explaining.

The objection to the idea that natural selection could operate on minute individual variations, drove De Vries to study the phenomenon of mutations, that is, of certain sudden and conspicuous variations which were alleged to have produced, in a single step, veritable new species.

But the sporadic occurrence of this phenomenon and the important part that atavistic phenomena seemed to play in it, and the small importance which consequently it was possible to attribute to it as a factor in evolution, impelled other scientific men to prefer the " Orthogenetic " theories of Nägeli and Eimer. These theories assumed a tendency of the germ-plasm (always supposed to possess a " Weismannian " continuity) to become gradually modified by its own internal conditions, and so to give rise to a phylogenetic evolution which would be equally independent of the direct action of the environment in the Lamarckian sense and of its indirect action in the Weismannian sense.

But as these orthogenetic theories proved equally incapable of explaining how an evolution, exclusively determined by internal conditions, could succeed in giving rise to organisms so well adapted to their environment and to their functions, biologists encountered again the old dilemma now brought more sharply than ever into prominence, viz., " Either natural selection as sole factor in evolution " or " the co-operation with it of the factor of the inheritability of acquired characters." The consciousness of this dilemma, along with the undermining of the faith in the exclusive importance of natural selection, led the most sceptical to give a more favourable consideration to the Lamarckian doctrine.

Experiments, observations and arguments in support of this doctrine increased in number. The conviction began to dawn in many minds that it had been a kind of collective scientific madness to reject a theory which threw such a brilliant light on all the fundamental problems of evolution which, without it, were totally inexplicable. But along with this conviction, which became more wide-spread and more firmly based, there grew up a painful appreciation of the formidable problem involved in the attempt to elucidate the mechanism of this kind of hereditary transmission.

This problem, this enigma, was the secret and powerful motive which, admitted or not, consciously or sub-consciously drove a whole army of bold researchers, following the footsteps of Wilhelm Roux, to busy themselves with all that series of observations and experiments comprised under the title " The mechanics of the development of the organism."

As, however, the number of minute observations on the manner of the succession of embryonic stages in widely different species became increased as a result of the study of " developmental mechanics," the marvellous phenomenon of the recapitulation of phylogeny by ontogeny stood out in ever clearer prominence. This phenomenon, which was discovered by Fritz Muller, but which had been particularly elucidated by Haeckel and which was generally known as Haeckel's " fundamental law of biogenesis ", had always been regarded as one of the strongest arguments in favour of evolution, but now, in the light thrown on it by the theory of the inheritability of acquired characters, it assumed a new aspect and one of fundamental importance, that is, it was seen to be a *mnemonic phenomenon.*

In fact Haeckel himself and Butler, Orr and Cope, asked what meaning could be assigned to this repetition, however abridged, of phylogenetic stages during ontogeny, other than that it was evidence that living substance *remembered* all the modes of being through which the species had passed as a result of the continual acquisition of new characters superimposed on the old.

Thus we see how, in spite of the vagueness which this mode of speech involves, the way was prepared for another theory still more comprehensive and remarkable which was put forward for the first time by Hering in 1870 at a meeting of the Academy of Vienna under the title of " Ueber das Gedächtniss als eine allgemeine Funktion der organischen Materie," according to which memory is the universal and fundamental function of all living substance. This was the theory which Semon adopted in his work " Die Mneme als erhaltendes Prinzip in Wechsel des organischen Geschehens," and which he developed still more widely, supporting it by a large series of facts which showed the deep-seated analogy which could be traced between biological phenomena in general and those of biological development in particular on the one hand, and on the other hand those of memory in the narrower sense.

Everyone can see what a magnificent synthesis of biology and psychology, that is of two out of the four or five main sub-divisions of human knowledge, would be effected if this affirmation of deep un-suspected analogies between vital and mnemonic phenomena could be substantiated, for it would enable us to conceive these latter as constituting the fundamental substratum and essence of all life.

Cellular specialisation in virtue of which each cell responds in its normal manner, even when it is excited by stimuli of widely different character from those to which it is accustomed, the transmissibility of acquired characters and the ontogenetic develop-ment of organisms, the innate instincts of animals, pyschic phenomena of whatever nature from simple memory up to their highest manifestation in logical reasoning, which is only a complex variety of memory, all these phenomena, thanks to the mnemonic sub-stratum which can be detected in all of them, may be considered as merely very different manifestations of one and the same fundamental phenomenon.

Even assimiliation, that principal characteristic of living matter—that mystery which chemistry fails to solve—may not ask whether it also is anything more than an essentially mnemonic phenomenon ? For really, if we contemplate living substance which is continually undergoing decomposition in the so-called processes of organic destruction which accompany functional activity, and which is reproduced during so-called periods of functional repose, of organic reconstruction and of assimilatory synthesis, which remains through all changes identical with itself, and is always ready, when it decomposes, to manifest again the same functional activities, must it not appear that it is the result of an activity of a mnemonic nature ? Moreover, one can see that it is just because assimilation is itself a mnemonic phenomenon that all other vital phenomena are likewise of a mnemonic nature.

But at this point a formidable problem arises. The comparison of general vital phenomena with mnemonic phenomena, notwithstanding the deep analogies which it discloses, cannot avoid appearing forced, even if it does not become reduced to a mere metaphor, if one ignores the real nature of mnemonic phenomena properly so called. For these phenomena, namely, ordinary psychic memory, belong to a category of phenomena less general and more complex than vital phenomena, for every manifestation of psychic memory is certainly a vital phenomenon whilst the opposite is not true ; how then, it may be asked, can mnemonic phenomena be used to explain vital phenomena ? Nevertheless the analogies between the two types of phenomena are so evident that the comparison of one with the other irresistibly forces itself on the mind. We are therefore driven to enquire whether both classes of phenomena, i.e., vital and mnemonic in the narrower sense, might not be explicable by the assumption of a third still more general and elementary type of activity of which both might be merely two aspects or two special manifestations. It is easy to grasp the importance which would accrue to such a theory : such an elementary activity which it postulates would then serve as the ground of all vital phenomena, and would make the great mystery of life a little less obscure to us.

This question, however, will be considered in the chapters which follow. In the present chapter we have attempted merely to emphasize the fact that evolutionary doctrine through all the most varied attempts at its explanation, and in spite of the most acute theoretic differences, has led to mnemonic theories of development, which postulate as the basis of organic evolution, nay of life itself, a fundamental character similar to the mnemonic property, which is just that which discriminates, in the last resort, living matter from the inorganic world.

CHAPTER II

The three dilemmas of embryology. The first dilemma : Preformation or Epigenesis ? The second dilemma : Preformistic gemmules or non-representative materials ? The third dilemma : Nuclear specialisation or qualitatively equal nuclear division ? Nature of " plasmatic " action. Intercellular bridges and the circulation of nuclear energy throughout the whole developing organism. The plasmatic action of this irradiated nuclear energy. Correlations of development. Compensatory growths. " Development is merely the result of a series of unequal rates of growth localised in different places " (Wilhelm Roux). Facts and arguments in support of the theory that nuclear " plasmatic energy " is essentially of a nervous nature.

THE THREE DILEMMAS OF EMBRYOLOGY .

IN the study of the development of organisms biologists encounter three fundamental problems more or less mutually dependent, which can be formulated in the three following dilemmas, viz. :

(1) Is development effected by preformation or epigenesis ?

(2) Is the germ-plasm composed of preformistic gemmules or is it made up of substances which are altogether devoid of the power of representing and of determining each a single morphological character or a special process of development ?

38

(3) Is there specialisation of nuclei or is nuclear division qualitatively equal ?

A rapid analysis of each of these three fundamental problems will show us that it is a mistake to suppose that they can be adequately stated in the three alleged dilemmas.

I.—THE FIRST DILEMMA.

PREFORMATION OR EPIGENESIS ?

The first of these three problems, as everyone knows is this :

Does each portion of an embryo contain everything which is required to determine its further development except the materials necessary for its continued nourishment ; in other words : could each portion of an embryo if it were at a given moment detached from the remainder of the organism, and if it were placed in an environment suitable for its continued life, continue to develop as if it still formed part of the organism ; or is the development of each part of the organism, on the contrary, determined by the actions and reactions which all parts of the organism exert on each other during development ?

In the first case one would say that development was due to preformation, in the second alternative that it took place by epigenesis.

Stated thus the problem seems easy to solve, and yet we find that, whilst a whole series of facts contradict in the most absolute manner the idea of preformation, another series of facts are equally irreconcileable with the theory of epigenesis.

The most characteristic facts which contradict the idea of preformation can be briefly subsumed in the five following categories, the first of which comprises all cases of general regeneration whilst the four others include different types of special regeneration.

General Regeneration

This alone constitutes a strong argument against preformation. For instance : If the determinants of the leg which are presumably contained in the first indistinct rudiment of the limb at the beginning of its formation are distributed to its different parts during its development, whence does it derive the new determinants required for its regeneration ? Those who support " preformation " answer that all the determinants are not distributed during development, but that at each level of a developing member there remains a residue termed " reserve idioplasm ", which is ready to begin the regeneration of the part to which in ordinary growth it would give rise, as soon as that part is removed. But this explanation, which is after all little more than verbal, is rendered nugatory by the four cases of special regeneration already alluded to.

Regeneration sui generis, *ordinarily termed Post-generation*

This type of regeneration was observed by Roux in the half-embryos of the frog which he obtained by killing with a red-hot needle one of the first two blastomeres.

We shall discuss later the significance which is to be

attributed to the half embryos themselves. Here we shall merely indicate the course of the regeneration which takes place. In the injured blastomere, which has not developed at all, and which has remained adherent to the intact blastomere now developed into a normal half-embryo, there begins at a certain moment a process of dissemination of nuclei derived by division, either from the still surviving nucleus of the injured blastomere or from the nuclei of the developed germ layers of the half embryo or from both sources. This dissemination of nuclei causes a belated division of the cytoplasm of the injured blastomere into small cells which are, however, quite undifferentiated and show no traces of the typical morphological arrangement. But later a change supervenes and we can observe in the injured blastomere the formation of germ layers, using as materials these undifferentiated cells ; the process of the formation of these new layers appears to start from the germ layers belonging to the uninjured half of the egg, and gradually invades the injured half so that it comes about that this latter half is brought to the same stage of development as that which has been attained by the uninjured half. Here then we can clearly see the "plasmatic influence" exerted by the fully formed germ layers of the uninjured half of the egg on the cellular material in the injured half.

Regeneration by Different Methods from those followed in Ordinary Development.

As an instance of this we may cite the celebrated case of the lens of the newt's eye which, after being cut off, is regenerated by a proliferation from the edge of the double epithelial layer of the iris ; in a word, the lens which has an ectodermic origin since it is developed from the outer ectoderm of the head in the embryo, is regenerated from the epithelium of the iris which is the front edge of the retina. Here it is clearly impossible to postulate " reserve idioplasm," for this, *ex-hypothesi*, is situated in the path traversed by the organ in its normal development and cannot therefore be present in the different path followed by the process of regeneration.

Regeneration by Rearrangement.

We shall confine ourselves to the consideration of the regeneration of *Planaria maculata* as this constitutes the most typical instance of this phenomenon. Fragments of this worm obtained by transverse cuts will regenerate head and tail respectively by the formation of new cells. Once formed, however, the new head and the new tail do not continue to grow in length ; all the subsequent elongation of the body, on the contrary, takes place in the original fragment which is more deeply pigmented than the newly regenerated portions. In this part the old tissues become changed by rearrangement into new tissues which are specifically different. In the same way in animals regenerated from lateral fragments, removed from one or other side of the original longitudinal axis of symmetry, it often happens that the longitudinal axis of the new worm is situated in the old pigmented tissue. In this case again tissues belonging to the right side of the original animal, which were constituents of definite organs in it, come to lie on the left side of the regenerated animal, and enter into the composition of totally different organs from those of which they originally formed part. These are cases of regeneration by re-arrangement which prove, as Whitman justly remarks, that it is the whole organism which governs the formation and fate of cells and not the cells which govern the organism, as the "preformationists" would have us believe.

Regeneration with Shortened Development.

Everyone knows that the salamander regenerates its tail in the rounded adult form and that the tail does not pass through a flattened stage such as it exhibits in the larva, and that the shrimp regenerates its claw in the adult condition and that the regenerated claw does not pass through a stage in which it resembles the corresponding limb of the zoæa larva. These facts indicate that these regenerations are not caused by "reserve idioplasm," which would cause development passing through the same stages as those traversed in normal ontogeny, but that regeneration in these cases is due to the influence exerted on the regenerating part by the remainder of the organism. In fact, this influence when the organism is adult is certainly different from what it is when the organism is in an earlier developmental stage, and so it follows that regeneration must pass through stages different from those of normal ontogeny.

The foregoing is a rapid and incomplete summary of

the principal facts which alone suffice to demonstrate in the most absolute manner the inadmissibility of development by preformation. [1]

But other facts prove in a manner not less absolute the inadmissibility of the theory of epigenesis. In order to confine ourselves here to the briefest summary of these we shall mention only the frog half-embryo obtained by Roux and the experiments of Born.

It was, in fact, these half-embryos which induced Roux to put forward his celebrated working hypothesis of " mosaic development."

Since it is possible to obtain the normal development of either the right or left half of the animal or of its anterior or posterior portion, one is driven to conclude that each of the four quarters of the organism derived from one of the first four blastomeres is capable of developing quite independently of the rest and that consequently, so far as concerns these four main sub-divisions, the embryo has a mosaic constitution.

The experiments of Born in grafting portions of amphibian larvæ lead to the same conclusion. A larva of *Rana esculenta* for instance, from which the anterior portion of the head had been removed, was grafted on to the ventral surface of a complete larva. After a dozen days of development all the organs of the mutilated larva had developed completely and perfectly normally as far as the surface of amputation. The anterior part of another larva, cut off a little

[1] For a more complete account of the facts involved and a more adequate discussion of them see our work " On the Inheritance of Acquired Characters." English translation, The Open Court Publishing Co., London and Chicago, 1911. Chapter IV, Section 2, " Facts which compel us to reject the theory of preformation."

behind the beginning of the spinal cord and grafted on the abdomen of a complete larva, pursued the normal course of its development ; the mesoderm out of which the skull is formed was, at the time of the amputation, almost completely undifferentiated and yet, nevertheless, the cartilaginous trabeculæ, the quadrate cartilages with their covering of masticatory muscles, Meckel's cartilages with the labial cartilages of the lower lip, and the hyoid cartilage itself were formed just as well as if the head had continued to form part of a complete organism. That this result was not due to the fact that the development of such an important organ as the head was involved was proved by the fact that a tail grafted under similar circumstances likewise pursued a normal course of development. [1]

What conclusion can we draw from all the facts which have been cited ? Simply that the dilemma " preformation or epigenesis," from which until now biologists imagined that they could not free themselves, appears to be non-existent and that consequently we must seek some means of evading it.

A hypothesis which is capable of reconciling these apparently contradictory facts is that of " centro-epigenesis." According to this theory a " plasmatic influence," which governs development, radiates out from a special region of the organism termed the " central zone of development." So that, if a portion of this zone is situated in an embryonic fragment detached from the rest of the organism, this

[1] See the work cited Chapter IV, Section 1, " Facts which compel us to reject the theory of simple epigenesis."

fragment will be able to pursue its proper course of development. [1]

With this hypothesis there would be no further difficulty in explaining the half-embryos of Roux and the partial developments of Born. All the apparently contradictory results of experiments on the influence of the nervous system on development and regeneration are also easily explained if one assumes that the central zone of development in vertebrates is constituted by a portion or a given layer of the spinal cord extending throughout its entire length, for instance by the most internal peri-ependymal layer and in the first stages of development by those blastomeres and cells which later give rise to this layer. [2]

In a word, in the light of the centro-epigenetic hypothesis the development of multicellular animals is seen to be of the same nature as that of unicellular animals ; in these latter, as is proved by the experiments of cutting the animals into pieces, the presence of the nucleus, or at least a fragment of it, is necessary and also sufficient to allow of the complete regeneration of a separated portion of an individual ; and thus the nucleus acts as a true " central zone of development."

But before developing our hypothesis further it is advisable to examine the second of the dilemmas

[1] See in the work cited Chapter III, Section 1, " Phenomena which lead us to suspect the existence of a central zone of development."

[2] Cf. Eugenio Rignano. " Die Centro-epigenetische Hypothese und der Einfluss des Zentralnervensystems auf embryonale Entwicklung und Regeneration. Arch. für Entwicklungsmechanik der Organismen." Vol. 21, Heft 2.

mentioned above which have excited so much controversy amongst biologists.

II.—SECOND DILEMMA

IS THE GERM-PLASM MADE UP OF PREFORMISTIC GEMMULES OR DOES IT CONSIST OF NON-REPRESENTATIVE MATERIAL?

Let us notice to begin with that this second dilemma is not quite indissolubly connected with the first dilemma as might at first sight be supposed. Thus de Vries who, like Weismann, assumes that the germ-plasm is constituted of preformistic gemmules, assumes also in opposition to Weismann, that development is epigenetic in its nature, and although amongst so-called chemical theories of the development of the egg, which reject the view that the egg is composed of preformistic gemmules, there are some which affirm the epigenetic nature of development, there are, nevertheless, others which incline towards a " preformist " view of development. According to these latter the succession of different chemical processes on which the development of each part of the organism depends, goes on independently in that part without being influenced by the similar successions of other chemical processes which take place in the other parts.

We shall now indicate briefly the principal argument which has been advanced in support of the theory that the germ-plasm is composed of preformistic gemmules.

This argument consists in stating that it would be impossible without this theory to account for the facts of particulate inheritance. This at least is the view of all the supporters of " preformistic gemmules " from Darwin and Galton to De Vries and Weismann.

The phenomena of the mixed inheritance of characters from father and mother, the phenomena of atavism, the characters of hybrids, the phenomena of spontaneous variation, all combine to show that the most trivial characters of organisms can be inherited quite independently of all other ; and hence the hypothesis is naturally suggested that each of these characters is specially determined by a seed or germ which bears the same relation to this character, as the whole seed or germ sustains towards the whole organism.

It is certain that hypotheses like those of Spencer which assume that the germ-plasm is made up of a homogeneous substance, are incapable of accounting for this power of the independent hereditary transmission of particular characters ; they cannot explain why two individuals may differ from each other only in one special character localised in a single determinate position in the body.

The same failure is found in theories which assume that the germ-plasm is a mixture of different chemical substances, all of which are in action from the beginning of development. Indeed, even if we assume the existence of two germ-plasms of identical natures except as regards one of the numerous substances of which they are composed, if this substance begins to act from the first moment of development, its different effect will be manifested from the beginning on the whole developing organism, which will therefore differ slightly in all its parts and not merely in one limited part from the other organism in which this substance is replaced by another.

On the other hand, if for the sake of brevity we leave out of account all the other formidable objections which can be raised against the theory of preformistic gemmules, and if we, therefore, do not refer to the circumstance that according to this theory every cell, and indeed every one of the smallest portions of each cell, must have its own gemmule, there is an argument which is sufficient to prove in the most absolute way that the whole theory is untenable, and this argument is that if the " gemmules " are going to explain particulate inheritance, and it is only for this purpose that they have been introduced, it is necessary to suppose that they are connected together by a rigid framework. In this point Weismann is perfectly right in his controversy with De Vries.

Let us consider for instance the " zebra striping " which sometimes appears as an atavistic phenomenon in certain horses which are otherwise quite similar to the normal type of horse. This striping cannot be merely due to the presence in the germ -plasm of these horses of gemmules capable of producing what may be briefly termed white and black cells. The appearance of stripes depends on the fact that at the completion of development the white and black cells are arranged in a determinate way in a determinate place in the organism. We must suppose, therefore, that in the germ-plasm or nucleus of the fertilised egg these gemmules are arranged with respect to each other in a rigid structure so that as the nucleus divides

49

it is these gemmules and no others which come to lie in given positions in the organism so as to give rise to the corresponding cells in the right place.

Such a fixed connection between gemmules is, indeed, just what is assumed in the famous theory of Weismann on the structure of the germ-plasm.

But this theory of a rigid architecture of the gemmules collapses at once when subjected to even the most superficial critical examination. For if we assume such an architecture, it is incomprehensible how the germ-plasm, after having grown in bulk, could divide and continually give rise to new germ-plasms which retain the same structural arrangement.

On this theory the course of development should be rigidly determined ; and this is irreconcilable with the great capacity for adaptation which organisms possess not only in their adult state, but also during the course of their developments ; that is made perfectly clear by all the phenomena of teratology. Development should take place according to the " preformist " plan and we have seen that the best established facts contradict in the most absolute manner the theory that development is of a " preformist " nature.

And so convincing arguments, of which we have set forth only the most important, force us to reject the theory of preformistic gemmules. At the same time no less important facts and arguments force us equally, as we have seen, to reject both the views that the germ-plasm is of a homogeneous nature or that it is composed of a mixture of different chemical substances all of which enter into action from the beginning of development.[1]

Therefore, the second dilemma from which biologists have imagined that they could not escape appears on closer examination to be of very dubious reality, and the suspicion arises that in this case also we might have recourse to an intermediate theory. Such a theory might be as follows : Let us suppose that the germ-plasm is composed of a number of elements of " specific potentiality," that is to say, if I may so express myself, of a number of elementary accumulators of a hitherto undefined " vital energy " which, perhaps, might be nervous energy ; these accumulators might be capable in discharging themselves not of giving back this form of energy indifferently in all the multifarious specific variations of which this energy is capable (as do electric accumulators in respect of electrical energy, all intensities of which can be given as discharges by the same accumulator), but of giving back each only a certain specific variety of this energy. Let us further suppose that these potential elements, which are at first contained in the nucleus of the fertilised egg and afterwards in the nuclei which make up the central zone of development, are discharged one after the other in a fixed order from the moment when the egg begins to segment until the adult state is attained, each of these discharges initiating and controlling a corresponding phase of the process of

[1] For the further description and discussion of the facts and arguments for and against the theory of " preformistic germs " see the work cited, Chap. V, sections 3 and 4, " Inadmissibility of a homogeneous germinal substance and inadmissibility of preformistic germs."

development itself. These accumulators would be preformistic gemmules *sui generis*. Instead of being determinants or representatives of different parts of the organism considered apart from each other, they would be determinants or representatives of each stage in ontogeny ; but they would be this solely in consequence of the fact that each, entering into activity after its predecessors, would find the organism in a state corresponding to the ontogenetic stage immediately preceding, and would consequently stimulate the organism to develop until it reached the next stage in ontogeny.

In this way, whilst one would no longer have to encounter the formidable objections which can be raised against the theory of preformistic gemmules, one could explain, and in this case without any difficulty, all the phenomena of particulate inheritance for which " preformistic gemmules " have been hitherto considered indispensable.

For instance if we consider the case of two embryos which have already nearly attained the adult condition, and which up till now have remained absolutely identical in their characters, and if we suppose that in one of them a new " specific potential element " suddenly comes into activity which is either absent in the other or represented there by a different element, and if in virtue of its peculiar specific variety this new element can only act on a special part of the body, then the two organisms might absolutely resemble each other in all their other characters and differ from one another only in one character localised in a single region of the body.

THE CENTRO-EPIGENETIC HYPOTHESIS

So we could explain all the varied phenomena of the independent inheritance of particular characters, and so render futile the principal argument in favour of the existence of preformistic gemmules, which Weismann considered to be demonstrative and absolutely irrefutable.

THE THIRD DILEMMA

IS THERE SPECIALISATION OF NUCLEI OR IS NUCLEAR DIVISION QUALITATIVELY EQUAL ?

Both those who oppose and those who support the doctrine of nuclear specialisation have thought it necessary to bring this dilemma into prominence because the qualitatively equal division of nuclei and nuclear specialisation have been considered to be two incompatible things. For if each nucleus, in dividing, gives rise to two daughter nuclei which are qualitatively alike, then, so runs the argument, all the nuclei of the adult organism must be like not only to each other, but also to the nucleus of the fertilised egg, whence all have been derived by successive nuclear divisions.

Now in this case also a whole series of facts and arguments may be adduced in favour of the equality of nuclear division, and another series of facts and arguments may be brought forward in support of nuclear specialisation.

The principal facts and arguments in favour of the equality of nuclear division are well known. It will be sufficient to mention in the briefest possible manner the most important of these which are as follows :

(1) *Isolation and displacement of blastomeres.*

So far as concerns the isolation of blastomeres everyone is familiar with the experiments of Chabry on ascidians, of Wilson on amphioxus, of Herbst on the sea-urchin, of Driesch on *Echinus microtuberculatus*, of Raffaele Zoja on medusæ, not to speak of others.

These experiments have demonstrated in an unanimous way that in all eggs in which the nutritive yolk or deutoplasm is neither too abundant, too dense, or too viscous, each of the isolated blastomeres, sometimes even one of the first 8, 16 or 32 blastomeres, is capable of giving rise to a complete embryo normal in every respect, but naturally of proportionately reduced size. In a similar way experiments on the displacement of blastomeres, experiments in which the spherical mass made up of the first blastomeres is squeezed between two glass plates, and so deformed in shape, have shown that when the upper plate is removed and a new mass of blastomeres is obtained in which the mutual positions of the different blastomeres have been completely modified, nevertheless a perfectly normal individual develops from this mass. These experiments also therefore demonstrate the equivalence of the different blastomeres amongst themselves up as far as the stage of the morula.

(2) *Double Monsters Originating from a Single Egg.*

Under this head we may mention the double gastrulæ obtained by Wilson from the egg of

Amphioxus, by slightly displacing the first two blasto-meres with respect to one another, and the double monsters obtained by Oscar Schulze from the eggs of the frog by inverting the slides between which the eggs were compressed immediately after the first two blastomeres had been formed. These experiments, which are essentially similar to those in which blasto-meres are isolated, confirm the results given by these latter.

(3) *Single Embryo arising from the fusion of two Blastulæ.*

It was Morgan who observed the spontaneous fusion of two blastulæ of Sphærechinus. The two blastulæ gave rise to a single blastula from which an entirely normal larva developed.

All these experiments on the isolation and displace-ment of blastomeres, on the production of double monsters from a single egg and on the development of a single individual as result of the fusion of two blastulæ with one another, constitute the most direct, tangible and irrefutable proof that one could desire, that all the nuclei of the first blastomeres are equivalent to each other and to the nucleus of the fertilised egg which is their common mother.

To these experiments on the earliest stages of development may be added others relating to the adult state of the lower organisms. We know, for instance, that any small piece of a hydra or of a medusa will transform itself without any increase in size into an entire individual of proportionately reduced dimensions.

At first sight this case seems to fall—and sometimes really falls—into the category of regeneration by the rearrangement of tissues, such as we have met with, for instance, in Planaria. However, when we take into consideration the minuteness and almost un-differentiated character of some of these pieces, many authors are inclined to think that the restitu-tion of the complete animal from such small fragments ought rather to be interpreted as a new process of development which is traversed anew from its first beginnings in consequence of the germinal properties retained by the fragment or by the nuclei in it.

In the same way we know that fragments of the leaves of *Begonia phyllomaniaca* planted in earth in a moist atmosphere give rise to small plants situated at the cut end of each nervure of the leaf.

From these facts we must consequently infer that the nuclei of cells, which certainly in the case of hydra as well as in that of the leaf of begonia per-formed some special somatic function in the original organism, retain nevertheless also all their germinal powers.

Nevertheless, in spite of all the experiments which we have mentioned, and of many other similar ones which seem to bear unanimous witness in favour both of the qualitatively equal character of nuclear division and of the fact that in the lower animals and in plants some of the somatic nuclei of the adult retain all their germinal powers, it is undeniable that the great majority of biologists continue to support the defenders of nuclear specialisation, who assert that the nuclei of cells histologically specialised and different from one another are also specialised and different from one another.

Why do the opinions of the majority, in spite of everything, incline in favour of nuclear specialisation ?

This is due to the fact that in many cases the nuclei, like the cells of the same organism, appear to be morphologically different from one another, that is to say that they appear to our eyes to differ from one another in certain peculiarities of their structure, of their processes of division, etc. At the same time chemical analysis seems to confirm the theory of a difference of composition between nuclei of different tissues.

But there is above all the very strong argument, and it is the principal one, deduced from the fact that the nucleus, as appeared to be fully established, is the portion or organ of the cell which for the greater part, or almost exclusively, determined the specificity or the various specificities of each cell. Consequently cells histologically different from one another, that is, cells which manifest specifically different physiological characters, could only be conceived of as provided with nuclei specifically distinct.

It is sufficient to consider that, if the hypothesis of nuclear specialisation is rejected, we must regard the nuclei of all the nervous centres as qualitatively equal to each other and to the nuclei of the other tissues !

To sum up, we see in this case also, as in those of the two dilemmas which we have previously considered, that there is a whole series of facts and arguments which support the view that nuclear division is qualitatively equal, and another large series in favour of the hypothesis of nuclear specialisation.[1]

Whence it follows that this dilemma, which until now has seemed inevitable to biologists, can have no more real existence than the two previous ones, and we must therefore seek some intermediate view which will reconcile the opposite sides of this question.

The first intermediate hypothesis which suggests itself to the mind is as follows :

Let us assume that nuclear division is qualitatively equal, in a word let us assume that each nucleus in dividing gives rise to two daughter nuclei similar to itself, and that consequently in its first division the nucleus of the fertilised egg gives rise to two nuclei similar to itself, each containing all the elements of the germ-plasm ; let us assume further that the same thing takes place when the nucleus of each of the first two blastomeres divides so as to produce the nuclei of the first four blastomeres, and so on, but that later, as development proceeds, other elements, which we shall term " somatic," are gradually added to the primary elements of the germ-plasm, as a consequence of the different position successively occupied by the nucleus in question, of the relations which develop between the nucleus and its neighbours and of the somatic functions which it assumes in consequence of its relations to its neighbours and of other similar circumstances. These " somatic "

[1] For the complete description and discussion of the facts and arguments for and against nuclear specialisation, see in the work cited, Chap. III, Section 2, " Hypotheses of the structure of the germinal substance."

elements which, like the primary germinal elements, possess the character of "specific potentiality," which we have explained in the preceding section, will come to be gradually deposited only in those nuclei which are outside the assumed "central zone of development," from which plasmatic action proceeds, and at first, in the earlier stages of development, they will be merely added to the primary germinal elements. Nevertheless, as development proceeds to later stages, these "somatic" elements, as they increase in number or in bulk in a measure depending on the nature of the organism or on the particular tissue to which they belong, will finally, in the struggle for space and nutrition, gradually displace the primary germinal elements.

In the lower animals and in many plants this complete substitution of somatic for germinal elements will not take place, at least in some tissues, and as a result of this fact germinal elements in an inactive state will continue to survive along with somatic elements in full functional activity ; with the consequence that these germinal elements will always be ready to initiate development, when exceptional circumstances permit them to become active.

If we now sum up our whole discussion on the three dilemmas, we see that, if we examine them without any preconceived ideas, of these three, on which biologists have vainly debated until now, not one will stand critical examination, but that in place of each of them it is possible to sketch an intermediate hypothesis capable of reconciling apparently contradictory facts, which precisely on account of this appearance of opposition have given rise to the dilemma.

It remains to be shown, as indeed must have already become evident to not a few of our readers, that these three intermediate hypotheses, with which we have solved the three corresponding dilemmas, can be combined and harmonised so as to form a single hypothesis to which we have already given the name of "centro-epigenesis." But before doing this it seems advisable to stop a moment to study as succinctly as possible what can be the nature of this "plasmatic" activity which, proceeding from the central zone, exerts its influence at every moment on each part of an organism in process of development.

The Nature of Plasmatic Action.

First of all we must examine rapidly the part played in this plasmatic action by the nuclei and by the intercellular protoplasmic bridges. Pfeffer has shown at the same time the importance of the protoplasmic filaments which join the protoplasm of one cell to that of its neighbour for the *transmission* of "plasmatic" action, and the importance of the nuclei for the *generation* of this plasmatic action.

He has shown that if the protoplasmic body of a cell be detached from the cell wall by plasmolysis, and if this body be then divided into two parts, one containing the nucleus and one devoid of nucleus, the nucleated portion will form a new cell-wall, which the enucleated portion is unable to do. But if this enucleated portion remains in connection with the nucleated portion by a thread of protoplasm, however thin, then it, too, will form a new cell-wall.

Pfeffer then made a preparation in which a mass of protoplasm devoid of nucleus and of cell-wall remained in contact with an uninjured cell by means of the protoplasmic filaments which normally unite two neighbouring cells with each other. He showed that in this case also the enucleated fragment formed a cell-wall round itself. He even succeeded in obtaining a chain of enucleated protoplasmic fragments connected with each other by protoplasmic bridges, of which the terminal member was a protoplasmic mass containing a nucleus, and he observed that in this case the formation of the new cell-wall took place centrifugally, that is to say that it was first formed round the piece nearest to the nucleated portion, and then successively round the fragments successively further removed from this.

This second experiment of Pfeffer would alone suffice to justify the hypothesis of a circulation throughout the organism of a particular form of energy which must be of the same nature as the discharges or stimulations proceeding from the nuclei.

It is, indeed, exceedingly probable that this nuclear stimulation which is transmitted from the nucleated cell along protoplasmic bridges to the enucleated fragment, is equally transmitted when this fragment has itself a nucleus, and even when it is a complete normal cell. This consideration leads us to assume that, wherever protoplasmic bridges exist, the various nuclear discharges unite along these bridges so as to give rise to a veritable tide of nuclear energy which floods the whole network of these protoplasmic bridges, a network of which the nodal points are constituted by the nuclei themselves.

If we grant the universal occurrence of these intercellular bridges connecting together all the cells of all the tissues at every period of development, beginning with the stage of the first blastomeres, we are led to regard it as very probable that this distribution of nuclear energy at every instant continues from the beginning of development up to and throughout the adult condition, and penetrates the entire organism.

This hypothesis of a circulation of nuclear energy throughout the entire organism, and consequently in each particular tissue, is supported by the following celebrated experiment of Siegfried Garten. He had a small disc of skin about 1 cm. in diameter cut out from his arm. Without uniting the edges of the wound he covered it with an aseptic bandage, and left it to heal. When the wound was almost completely closed—leaving only a small disc of about 1.75 mm. in diameter in the centre uncovered—he cut away the new skin which had been formed, and examined it under the microscope. He then observed that this skin consisted of concentric zones of cells of different aspects. In one of these rings, which contained the largest cells, the intercellular bridges were extraordinarily well developed, and it was only in this zone that nuclear divisions were to be seen.

If we assume for a moment that there is a continuous flow of nuclear energy across the intercellular bridges, the remarkable development of these bridges in one of the zones of cells surrounding the wound receives an immediate explanation.

For this nuclear current, which previously passed through the intra-cellular filaments and intercellular bridges of the cells belonging to the little disc of skin which was cut out, would after the excision find its normal paths blocked, and would be constrained to flow around the wound, and so would increase the amount of current which normally traversed this region. This increased current would create for itself the means of passage, either by increasing the diameter of the protoplasmic bridges or by augmenting their number.

If we recollect that it is precisely in the zone where these bridges are best developed, and only in it that we meet with nuclear divisions, we see that we can learn something further from this experiment, namely, that the increase in the amount of the nuclear current exerts a trophic influence on the growth in bulk of the living substance, as a consequence of which there is a great proliferation of nuclei in its path.

This is extremely interesting, because it enables us, hypothetically at least, to account for the differences in rate of growth which are encountered in different parts of the same tissue, and in different tissues of the same organism, by differences in the amount of the nuclear current.

But now we must pass to the question of the probable nature of this energy which so far we have denominated by the term nuclear. If we recall the fact that in unicellular organisms amongst the direct and indirect effects of nuclear stimulation, there are some which take the form of contractions of vibratile cilia and of consequent movements; if we remember further that even in higher animals in which in the adult condition the ultimate cause of movement is beyond all possible doubt nervous energy, movements nevertheless begin in the earliest embryonic stage, as is proved by the free-swimming blastulæ and gastrulæ of all the animals whose eggs develop freely in the water; if we consider that all plants manifest the phenomena of contraction as a result of irritation, and that the most sensitive plants have better developed intercellular bridges than those that are less sensitive; if we take account of all these facts and of many others too numerous to cite here, it will not appear too daring to advance, as a purely provisional hypothesis, that nuclear discharges are of the same nature as nervous discharges. If this is so, the flow of nuclear energy which traverses the entire organism and penetrates every part of it will be nothing but nervous energy.

Hertwig himself has lent the great support of his authority to this view. He expresses himself as follows: " It is probable that in comparison to the conduction of stimuli by nerves, the transmission of nuclear stimulation by means of protoplasmic filaments is much less rapid and intense, but for that reason it is more continuous and, by reason of its duration, more efficacious."

On this view the nervous fibres and fibrillæ would be fundamentally nothing else than intercellular bridges uniting the nerve cells to the other tissues, and the continuous distribution of nervous energy throughout the organism would be effected not only by the close network formed by the intercellular bridges, but also by all the network made up of the nerves, fibres and fibrillæ of the nervous system.

Before we proceed further we must emphasise the fact that this hypothesis of a continuous circulation of nervous energy is capable of being applied not only to animals but also to plants.

First of all we have the experiments of Pfeffer referred to above, which were done on the cells of plants. We know besides that in recent years several scientists, notably Francis Darwin of Cambridge, Haberlandt of Graetz, and Francé of Munich, have studied the interesting phenomena of the sensitiveness and movements of plants ; the results obtained by these researchers demonstrate that plants in general are sensitive, and we have already alluded to the fact that the most sensitive possess better developed intercellular bridges ; moreover, in plants, as in animals, it is necessary to recognise a region of perception and a region of movement more or less distant from one another between which a transmission occurs, which we have every reason to suspect of being nervous in nature. There is indeed a " physio-psychology of plants " which is growing and establishing its right to be recognised as parallel with the physio-psychology of animals.

If then we assume for any given animal or plant in the adult condition or in any stage of its development that this nervous circulation is in operation, we have only to suppose that this is subject during ontogeny to continual changes in its mode of distribution in order to obtain a probable explanation of a whole host of developmental phenomena. We shall confine ourselves here to mentioning the principal of these, which are as follow :

(1) *Phenomena of the correlation of development*, not to be confounded with correlation of functions properly so-called. They consist in the circumstance that certain portions of the embryo, even if distant one from the other and without any functional relation to one another, seem to exercise on one another a reciprocal influence which governs or aids in governing their respective development. The development of one is accelerated with that of the other, is retarded when the development of the other is retarded and its development ceases when the other ceases to develop. If now, given parts of the organism, even if widely separated from one another, belong to the same main branch of the general distribution of nervous energy, and if others of different origin become gradually wedged between the parts of the first branch, though they belong to another branch of the distribution of nervous energy, we can understand how the mutual dependence of the parts belonging to the first branch on each other, and of those belonging to the second branch also on each other, can be brought about in the almost complete absence of any discoverable influence exercised by the parts of the first branch on those of the second branch.

(2) *Compensatory growth of organs not yet arrived*

66

at the stage of functioning. These have been studied chiefly by Ribbert and his pupils, and such are the discovery that the excision of a testis or of a mammary gland, even in the embryonic condition, stimulates the growth of its fellow. In this case we need only assume that a main branch of the system of distribution of nervous energy bifurcates, exerting its trophic influence on both testes and on both mammary glands during their development, in order to explain why if one of the forks of the bifurcating path is blocked, the whole nervous current is constrained to pass down the other, thereby exercising on it a proportionately greater trophic influence.

But it is after all the most general phenomenon of ontogeny which is in certain aspects most clearly explicable by this theory of a distribution of trophic nervous energy. Development at bottom is only, as everyone knows, the result of the unequal distribution of growth (Roux). The widest possible variety of form is produced by means of the most simple and monotonous system conceivable, viz., stimulation of cellular proliferation at a given point in a cellular layer more than in neighbouring points, so that the extra cells thus produced are forced to bend outwards (evagination) or inwards (invagination). We need only assume a continual change in the general system of distribution of nervous energy in order to understand this continual shifting of the points of more intense trophic activity.

The ontogenetic processes of involution (absorption) are typical examples of this shifting, as for instance the involution of the tail of the tadpole. We find at the beginning of metamorphosis an atrophy and degeneration of the skin, spinal cord and of nervous and muscular fibres. It is not a case, let us note, of a senile atrophy or of one brought on by cessation of functioning, but a physiological atrophy of pre-eminently young tissues. And since at this period the animal takes little or no food, whilst other organs undergo a sudden and rapid development, the substance of the degenerating tissues is absorbed and carried away by the lymphatic and vascular channels in order to be used for the building up of other organs which are now in course of rapid development. All this process seems to be explicable on the assumption that the nervous energy formerly distributed to certain regions has abandoned them completely and has been diverted to others.

But if we assume that normal ontogeny, in so far as it is made up of a series of shiftings of the regions of intense growth, is the result of continual changes of the general system of distribution of trophic nervous energy in the embryo, we have still to explain why this distribution continually changes during the whole development.

This will compel us to recapitulate in a few words our " centro-epigenetic " hypothesis of which the main features have been sketched in the preceding pages. To do this will be the task of the next chapter.

CHAPTER III

THE HYPOTHESIS OF A PLASMATIC ACTION RADIATING FROM A CENTRE AS THE BASIS OF A MNEMONIC THEORY OF DEVELOPMENT—(*continued*)

The three dilemmas arising out of the study of the development of organisms can be solved by the hypothesis of a plasmatic action radiating from a centre (centro-epigenesis). The central zone of development from which the influence radiates. The accumulation of specific deposits in the nuclei which make up the central zone. The gradual specialisation of the nuclei which lie outside this zone. The successive ontogenetic stimuli which give rise to development are only the reproduction, by internal causes, of the physiological activities which have been produced in the past by the functional stimuli to which preceding generations became adapted. Each new stage added to the phylogenetic history deposits as its representative one more specific potential element in the germ-plasm. This power of specific accumulation and the centro-epigenetic nature of development explain the recapitulation of phylogeny by ontogeny and supply us with a clue to the mechanism of the inheritance of acquired characters. The theory of centro-epigenesis solves all the difficulties which are involved in other mnemonic theories of development.

THE critical examination to which in the last chapter we have subjected the three dilemmas raised by the study of embryology, has led us to regard it probable that these three dilemmas could be solved by substituting for them the three following intermediate hypotheses :

(1) That the " plasmatic " action proceeds from a special part of the organism termed the " central zone of development."

(2) That the germ-plasm, that is the nucleus of the

69

fertilised eggs, is made up of a certain number of specific potential elements or elementary accumulators of a vital energy (and we are now able with the best chances of hitting the truth to conceive of this as nervous energy) which are capable by discharging themselves of giving rise not to discharges of this vital or nervous energy in general, but each only to a definite specific discharge of this energy ; and that these accumulators become active one after another in a definite order from the first beginning of development until its completion.

(3) That in the nuclei outside the central zone, which come to lie in cells which are histologically specialised, there gradually become added to the original specific potential elements of the germ-plasm, which are transmitted entire from nucleus to nucleus by qualitatively equal division, other specific potential elements different from the primitive ones, but of the same nature, which, increasing in number or bulk, gradually displace the primitive elements and substitute themselves for these. This process, which is due to limitations of space and nutrition, can, in the majority of cases, proceed to the complete substitution of the one series for the other, and so lead to a veritable specialisation of nuclei.

Once we assume, for reasons adduced in the preceding chapters, that the " plasmatic " action is caused by a general system of distribution of trophic nervous energy, we find, as every reader on reflection will see for himself, that these three hypotheses can be fused and harmonised in a single organic hypothesis.

The only point which deserves special discussion is the way in which certain nuclei originally qualitatively equivalent to the rest, gain the control of the others and come to constitute the central zone of development and so condemn these outer nuclei to become gradually reduced to somatic nuclei.

But the way in which this occurs will become clear when we take into account the following consideration. At the beginning of development, from the commencement of the segmentation of the egg until the morula or even the blastula stage is attained, when the nuclei are still all qualitatively equal to one another and to the nucleus of the egg whence they have been derived, we may consider these nuclei as all ready to begin the same kind of plasmatic action, at least in the only case which for the sake of simplifying the problem we shall consider here, viz., where all the blastomeres are equivalent to one another.

This condition of affairs, however, can only last until the time when the modification produced by the development is no longer uniform for all the parts of the embryo, as when an invagination, or similar process, is brought about, for then the nuclear energies cannot continue to operate in exactly the same manner in all the cells. From this period those of the nuclei which possess, whether by the accident of better nutrition or for any other accidental reason, a greater amount of potential energy than the others, even if their superiority in this respect is very slight (perhaps in meroblastic eggs, those which occupy a more favourable position than others), must gain the control of the latter and continue alone the process of discharging successive specific germinal energies, which they now inhibit in all besides themselves.

From this time the remaining nuclei, not allowed to constitute the central zone of development, and now under the control of the nuclei which make up this zone, become more and more specialised, because the tide of successive specific energies now passes through them, following the system of distribution determined at each moment by the corresponding activity of the central zone.

For each new potential element which enters into activity in the nuclei of the central zone will disturb the dynamic equilibrium of the general system of the distribution of nervous energy which has become established by the action of the preceding element, and will cause it to change to a new state of equilibrium corresponding to the next stage of development.

As one element after another of the central zone enters into activity, the development of the organism will traverse all its successive stages, and it will only cease when the action of these elements is completed, because the disturbing action of the central zone on the general dynamical equilibrium of the organism will then come to an end, and the definite equilibrium of the adult stage will be established.

Such are, briefly described, the general outlines of the centro-epigenetic hypothesis, constructed by fusing and harmonising the three intermediate hypotheses which were put forward to solve the three fundamental dilemmas mentioned above. Now, although this hypothesis has only been here sketched in baldest outline, it can immediately be seen to have one quality of supreme importance, viz., it can supply an explanation of the process of the hereditary transmission of acquired characters, by meeting the last serious objection to this view behind which the Neo-Darwinians, with Weismann at their head, could entrench themselves in their brave and desperate fight against Neo-Lamarckism, which in all other respects might be considered as triumphant. For just in the same way as, till now, the disturbing action of the central zone had interrupted the just-formed dynamic equilibrium and caused the passage of the organism from one ontogenetic stage to the next, so when the adult stage has been attained, each lasting change of functional stimulus, or of functional activity which results therefrom, will again upset what would otherwise have been the final condition of dynamic equilibrium, and cause the organism to pass to a new phylogenetic stage.

The alteration in the distribution of nervous energy which will result from this change will bring it about that through every cell of the organism or through each cell of a given region of the organism, a new current of energy will pass, specifically different in the different cells, and different also from the current which formerly traversed the same path. In each nucleus of these cells a new specific potential element will then be formed and deposited and so added to the number of the pre-existing elements.

But all these elements, new as well as old, which are deposited in the somatic nuclei, will be lost at the death of the individual, and only those will escape destruction which are deposited in the germ-plasm of the central zone. The only effect, therefore, of the lasting change of functional stimulus in the species will be the addition of a new potential element to the germ-plasm.

We must now investigate the way in which this new element acts during the ontogeny of the daughter organism. In order to explain this we shall have only to assume that the substance which constitutes each potential element, and which is capable of originating, when discharged, a single definite specific variety of nervous current, is, at the same time, the very same substance which this current can form and deposit, in order to explain how the new specific potential element, which has been deposited in the central zone of the parent organism, can, by entering into activity at the proper time in the central zone of the daughter organism, reproduce in this individual the same change which was caused in its parent by the action of the environment.

Thus the ontogenetic stimulus is merely a restitution or reproduction, by internal causes, of the functional stimulus or physiological reaction which is at first produced and can only be produced by the external medium. It follows also *that ontogeny is nothing but a continual adaptation of the embryo to successive modes of the activity of the central zone*, and that the fundamental law of biogenesis, viz., that ontogeny is a succinct repetition of phylogeny, appears to be the direct consequence of the mechanism of the hereditary transmission of acquired characters.

Even the acquisition of the most complex instincts

74

is therefore merely a special case of this transmission, and also sexual dimorphism, polymorphism in general, atavism, and a whole series of other more or less fundamental phenomena of development can thus receive their explanation. All these are points which must be already evident to most readers, but for the full elucidation of which we must refer to our work already cited several times.[1]

We may, however, add a few words in order to emphasise two characteristic consequences of the centro-epigenetic hypothesis.

The first is that this hypothesis is capable of explaining a " certain dose " of preformism, the existence of which seems to be placed beyond doubt by the results of certain experiments—results which have inflicted a mortal wound on the theory of simple epigenesis. We allude for instance (to name only the most typical) to the experiments of Braus, who transplanted the first undifferentiated rudiments of the fore and hind limbs of a toad to other positions on the same animal, and found that in their new positions they developed into typical adult members.

Certainly the results of these experiments do not justify the claim made by certain preformists, in spite of the repeated contrary results given by other similar experiments, and of a thousand other facts equally irreconcileable with their thesis, viz., that the same ontogenetic autonomy must then be true for any portion of the body, no matter how small, when separated from the rest. However, it cannot

[1] See Chap. VII, " The centro-epigenetic hypothesis : the explanation which it gives of the hereditary transmission of acquired characters."

be denied that the continued development of members separated from the rest of the body proves that they contained in themselves at the time of their amputation all that was necessary to determine their further development.

Now the centro-epigenetic hypothesis does not exclude the possibility that the early entry into activity of a series of specific potential elements of the central zone may leave such effects on certain portions of the body, that, even if these portions are removed at a certain moment from the direct action of the central zone, the development may continue as a sort of posthumous result of the activity of this zone. Something of this kind can be seen in the enucleated fragments of some infusoria, as for instance *Stentor cœruleus*. Although the nucleus is for infusoria as for unicellular animals in general a true and typical central zone of development, since without a nucleus no process of development or regeneration can be either begun or completed, yet Gruber has observed that if the animal showed at the time of the operation signs of spontaneous division, with rudiments of its peristomal band of cilia already appearing, the enucleated fragment would continue the development of this band, as a result of just this " posthumous action " of the now absent nucleus. This action can only be explained if we assume that a whole series of nuclear stimuli had already been emitted and had left their traces on the cell body, and it only remained to observe the slow development of these effects.

On the other hand we may ask how could the theory of simple epigenesis, in order to explain the results of these experiments of Braus, have recourse to a precocious entry into activity of a whole series of successive actions, which the remainder of the organism should have exerted on the amputated member ? These successive actions could only be produced by those modes of being of the remaining part of the organism which are realised after the occurrence of amputation, and would not for that very reason be possible before amputation.

The second consequence of the centro-epigenetic hypothesis which remains to be mentioned is that it makes it necessary for us to distinguish between *effective* and *apparent* germinal zone.

As we have already indicated everything leads us to believe—if we confine ourselves to organisms with a nervous system—that the central zone coincides with the least differentiated part of the nervous system. On the other hand, that which constitutes the central zone is just the germ-plasm, which remains always identical with itself throughout the entire development, in spite of the " plasmatic action " which it is continually exercising on the developing organism, and which would be transmitted unaltered from generation to generation were it not for the addition of elements resulting from the acquisition of new characters.

The central zone in vertebrates which, let us reiterate, is probably formed by the most internal layer of the spinal cord, would be the really *effective* germinal zone, that is the true place of the emission of germinal substance—just as, might we suggest, the marrow of the bones constitutes the place where the erythroblasts or embryonic red corpuscles of the blood are formed, whence they pass into the blood and are distributed by the circulation. The *apparent* germinal zone on the other hand, which is constituted by the genital organs, would only be—as these organs are in the old Darwinian hypothesis—the place for the reception, elaboration, and re-emission of the germinal substance, that is to say the place where this precious material is collected, which, by being taken up by certain cells selected by chance from thousands of others, and by being added to or substituted for the substance of the nuclei already in these cells, changes them from simple somatic into reproductive cells.

Is it perhaps the reception of germinal substance which constitutes the " maturation " of the reproductive cells ? Synapsis, that phenomenon recently discovered and still imperfectly investigated, in which the chromatin which will afterwards constitute the chromosomes of the egg and of the spermatozoon goes through the most complicated and mysterious changes, does it indicate the precise moment of the penetration of this germinal substance into a cell previously somatic or does it indicate the time immediately after this penetration when the germinal substance begins to instal itself in its new abode ?

To these questions, on which will depend in large measure the greater or less success that will accompany our hypothesis in the future, further research can alone give an adequate answer. We shall confine ourselves here to these brief remarks which we have thought it necessary to make, in order that along with the numerous and powerful arguments in favour of the

THE CENTRO-EPIGENETIC HYPOTHESIS (*cont.*)

centro-epigenetic hypothesis, we should not omit to mention the most important objection which might be raised against it.

THE MNEMONIC NATURE OF LIFE

Before completing this rapid and imperfect sketch of the centro-epigenetic hypothesis, it is necessary to show how it is related to other recent theories which seek to explain development and all the other characteristic phenomena of life by the fundamental mnemonic property of living substance, and how our theory may be regarded as the completion and final outcome of these theories.

As we have already stated in the first chapter, the phenomenon of the recapitulation of phylogeny by ontogeny, or the fundamental law of biogenetics, has always been considered to be of a mnemonic nature. Haeckel himself, Butler, Cope, Orr, if we consider only the principal exponents of this view, have seen at once, more or less vaguely, that this repetition of phylogenetic stages (however abridged) during ontogeny, is nothing but a manifestation of the memory retained by the living substance of all the modes of existence through which the species had passed in its continual endeavour to adapt itself to the successive changes of the environment.

In the celebrated address delivered before the Academy of Vienna, in 1870, Hering, under the suggestive title of "Ueber das Gedächtniss als eine allgemeine Funktion der organisierten Materie," made a daring step forward in maintaining that memory

79

is the general and fundamental function of living matter.

In his famous work entitled "Die Mneme als erhaltendes Prinzip in Wechsel des organischen Geschehens," Semon, as we know, took up and developed more fully Hering's proposition, adducing in its support a large number of facts which showed the deep analogy which existed between vital phenomena in general and those of ontogeny in particular, and the phenomena of memory in the stricter sense of the word. But the comparison of vital phenomena in general with memory, in spite of the deep resemblance between the two which it brings to light, can only appear artificial, and is even reduced to an innocent metaphor, if we do not take account of what memory in the narrower sense really is. For ordinary psychic memory belongs to a category of phenomena of a less general order and more complex than ordinary vital phenomena, since every manifestation of psychic memory is certainly a vital phenomenon, whilst the contrary is not true ; how then can memory be used to explain vital phenomena ?

Moreover mnemonic phenomena in the narrower sense are always " localised," whilst all " mnemonists " have completely ignored this fact when discussing the mnemonic nature of development.

Semon, for instance, who may be taken as a representative of this school, in order to surmount the difficulty of localisation, assumes that the effect of every stimulus, which acts on any given part of the body, diffuses throughout the organism, diminishing in intensity as it gets further from the point of incidence but remaining always identical in quality, so that proceeding from the zone where it exercises its maximum effect the stimulus will succeed in influencing and in " stamping an impression upon " all the cells of the body, including the reproductive cells and even all the small living components or " protomeres " of each cell. " Protomeres " or " plastidules " are old conceptions invented by Haeckel, which explain nothing, and indeed are devoid of all singificance. What meaning indeed could we assign to the statement that a complex visual impression was transmitted unaltered to the protomeres of the muscular fibres and the glandular cells, etc., or how could a local functional adaptation become spread over the whole organism ? [1]

It is just these difficulties which are obviated by the theory of centro-epigenesis.

Our theory surmounts the first difficulty, substituting for the explanation of vital phenomena by means of those of memory in the strict sense, a simpler hypothesis which assumes the existence of a more elementary and fundamental phenomenon of which vital phenomena and psychic memory are only two different aspects or special cases. We allude, of course, to the property which we have supposed to be characteristic of the specific potential elements of the nuclei both of germ-cells and somatic cells, viz., that each element in discharging itself gives rise to a nervous current of a definite specific character; and that the substance which produces this current is the same

[1] See Chapter V of this work, " The Mnemonic Theory of Semon."

substance which this current can and does in its turn deposit when acting as current of charge. This property confers on the specific potential elements or accumulators a true mnemonic nature.

Cellular specialisation in virtue of which each cell gives its proper and characteristic response even when excited by stimuli of a different character from those to which it is usually subjected ; the great law of the acquisition of habit to which all living substance is subjected ; the development of organisms ; the fundamental law of biogenetics or the recapitulation of phylogeny in ontogeny ; the transmissibility of acquired characters ; the inborn instincts of animals ; all these phenomena which suggest vaguely that they have some common basis, more or less analogous to memory, are seen, in the light of our hypothesis of specific nervous accumulators to be clearly and definitely nothing but so many manifestations or so many direct results of one and the same elementary phenomenon which we have now sharply defined.

Our theory surmounts likewise the second difficulty by localising phylogenetic memory in the central zone, constituted by the germ-plasm, and by supposing that the latter emits specifically the same effect in the opposite direction as that which the external stimulus has produced in it. It is then sufficient to assume, as we have seen, that this germ-plasm is situated in a definite part of the organism which is always the same, both when the body of the parent is exerting its action on its own germinal substance and when this germinal substance is acting upon the body of the embryo, in order to explain the succession of ontogenetic stages as the mnemonic repetition of phylogenetic stages.

But the theory of the specific accumulation of nervous energy does not exhaust its possibilities in explaining the fundamental mnemonic character of vital phenomena, and of all the consequences, direct and indirect, which flow from this elementary property. In the illumination of the light which it diffuses over the whole domain of biology, even the phenomena of assimilation, of the trophic action exerted by functional activity, and of the rejuvenescence caused by fertilisation appear a little less mysterious than before. These points we shall endeavour to make clear in the following chapter.

CHAPTER IV

THE ENERGETIC PROPERTIES OF BIOLOGICAL MEMORY

Short summary of our centro-epigenetic hypothesis. First provisional hypothesis of the energetic properties of nervous energy. The nervous accumulations have the property, found only in them, of producing the same specific variety of energy as that which caused their deposition. The two factors in energy, viz., capacity and intensity. The specific differences distinguishing two nervous currents might depend on differences in the capacity of their constituent elements. This might explain the exact correspondence between the specific variety of the current and the specific variety of accumulation. From this hypothesis also the laws of mnemonic association and of inhibition could be derived. Assimilation itself would then be seen to be a mnemonic phenomenon. The trophic influence of functional activity and the rejuvenescence produced by fertilisation would also receive an explanation. We could finally explain the universal tendency of life towards a limitless expansion.

(1) *Summary of the centro-epigenetic hypothesis.*

As we have seen in the preceding chapter, the essential part of our centro-epigenetic hypothesis can be summed up as follows :

The " plasmatic action " of the developing organism radiates out from a special region of this organism termed the central zone of development and made up of the germ-plasm.

The plasmatic action is due to successive modes of distribution or circulation of trophic nervous energy which is made up of all the nuclear excitations of all the embryonic cells.

These excitations flow together in the protoplasmic

84

bridges uniting the various cells with one another, being added to one another in the same path and split up along diverging paths, and the resulting system of nervous circulation penetrates the entire organism at each stage of the development and determines at every period its morphological and physiological condition.

The germ-plasm contained in the nucleus of the fertilized egg is made up of a large number of specific potential elements, that is to say, of a large number of elementary accumulators of nervous energy, which are able in discharging themselves to give rise, not to a current of undifferentiated nervous energy, as electric accumulators do for electric currents, but each to a definite specific variety of this nervous energy. These specific potential elements come into action one after the other from the beginning until the completion of development.

Each nervous current, each nervous excitation, whether it proceeds directly from a single nucleus or whether it results from the union or splitting up of several nervous currents, when it passes through another nucleus, even though this be a somatic one, deposits in it a " specific accumulation "—that is a substance which can originate by its decomposition exactly that kind of nervous current by the action of which it was deposited. Every nucleus, including somatic nuclei, may be supposed to be made up of numerous elementary accumulators similar in their general nature to those contained in the original nucleus of the germ-cell, but differing specifically from these and from one another.

The specific potential elements contained in the nucleus of the fertilised egg are transmitted unaltered from nucleus to nucleus as a consequence of the equality of nuclear division. But in those nuclei which as development proceeds are finally excluded from the central zone, and which come to lie in cells destined to become histologically specialised cells, there are gradually added new " somatic " specifically potential elements, in virtue of this power which each nervous current possesses of depositing a corresponding accumulation of itself. These "somatic" specific potential elements, increasing in number and in bulk, finally displace completely the primitive germinal elements and lead thus to a complete somatic specialisation of these nuclei.

If this hypothesis be accepted, let us consider how development should progress, beginning with the first segmentation of the egg.

In consequence of the equality of nuclear segmentation, the nuclei of the first blastomeres are all similar to each other and to the nucleus of the fertilised egg from which they were produced, and they will continue to be so at least up to the stage of the morula or of the blastula. These nuclei will therefore be all equally capable (especially if the blastomeres in which they lie are also similar to one another as is the case with holoblastic eggs) of exercising the same " plasmatic action " since each begins to discharge the same series of specific varieties of nervous energy.

But soon the moment will arrive when the new specific energies as they are discharged, are capable of producing an ontogenetic modification which is no longer uniform over the whole surface of a spherical blastula, as for instance an invagination. The entry into activity of the remainder of the specific energies cannot thereafter take place in all the blastomeres. From this time on those nuclei which in virtue of a better nutrition or of any other accidental circumstance possess a larger quantity of potential energy (or those, as in the case of meroblastic eggs, which occupy a more favourable position) will necessarily gain an advantage over the rest and will alone continue to discharge the successive specific energies a process which at first took place in all the nuclei, but which these favoured nuclei will now inhibit in all others but themselves.

From this time also the remaining nuclei which have been in this way excluded from the central zone and which are now under the control of those which constitute the central zone, will gradually become differentiated and specialised, for they will be constantly traversed by specific varieties of nervous energy, continually varying in character and amount according to the general system of circulation determined at each stage by the corresponding activities of the central zone. For every new specific potential element which becomes active in the nuclei of the central zone will upset the dynamic equilibrium of the general system of distribution of nervous energy which has been established as a result of the action of the previous element, and will so lead to the production of a new state of equilibrium corresponding to the next stage of development.

The germinal elements of the central zone will

enter into activity one after the other, and will cause the organism to pass through its successive stages of development, and this process will only cease when all the elements have entered into activity. Then the disturbing action of the central zone on the dynamic equilibrium of each ontogenetic stage will come to an end, and in this way the organism will reach a state of definite equilibrium—or " stationary state," as Ostwald terms it, which is the adult condition.

In the same way, however, as the disturbing action of the central zone was continually upsetting the equilibrium which had just been established and causing the organism to pass into a later stage of development, when the adult stage has been finally attained, each new external stimulus, or complex of stimuli which is not transient, in a word each persisting change in the action which the environment exerts on the organism, which, of course, induces a corresponding persisting reaction on the part of the organism, will have the effect of upsetting once more the dynamic equilibrium which would otherwise have remained fixed and definite. As a result, the organism will pass into a new physiological and morphological condition which will constitute its next phylogenetic stage.

Each of these physiologico-morphological states will be represented in the part of the organism occupied by the germ-plasm by a special type of nervous current, the peculiar characters of which will be a function and expression of the general system made up of the innumerable currents emitted by all the nuclei of the organism. This resultant nervous current will thus be the representative current of this particular phylogenetic stage.

The successive phylogenetic stages will thus each possess, in relation to the central zone constituted by the germinal substance, their representative currents, and each representative current will deposit its own specific accumulation representing the corresponding phylogenetic stage in the germ-plasm ; and this deposit will be capable in each new ontogeny of giving anew as discharge the same particular current which caused its deposition. We need only therefore assume that the germ-plasm is always situated in the same relative part of the organism, both when it is receiving and storing these currents and when it is emitting the same currents during ontogeny, to see that the organism during its development must pass through the whole series of physiologico-morphological states, through which the species passed during its evolution ; though, of course, this series may be more or less abridged according to the greater or less perfect manner in which the specific accumulations have been preserved. In the same way, it is only necessary that a single point of the membrane of a phonograph should reproduce all the modes of being through which it passed when it received a given series of auditory vibrations, in order that the whole membrane should traverse again all the extraordinarily complicated modes of being, which were originally produced by the action of the external world, and which are now reproduced by the action of a single internal point.

We thus see that the fundamental law of biogenetics, viz., the recapitulation by ontogeny of phylogeny is an immediate consequence of the process by which acquired characters are inherited.

Such is in its main outlines our centro-epigenetic hypothesis which, being founded entirely on the mnemonic property which we have assumed to be peculiar to vital phenomena, impels us to seek to put forward some hypothesis, even if it were only a purely provisional one, which would let us catch a glimpse of the dynamical foundations on which this mnemonic property is based.

(2) *First and provisional hypothesis of the energetic properties of nervous energy.*

We have seen that the recapitulation of phylogeny by ontogeny, which can be directly explained by our centro-epigenetic hypothesis, has from the beginning been regarded as a mnemonic phenomenon. Starting from this point, biologists have been gradually led, as we have already seen, especially in the works of Hering and Semon, to the position of regarding memory as the most general and fundamental function of all living matter.

All these comparisons of ontogeny and memory, these extensions to living substance in general of the mnemonic property, although based on certain very suggestive analogies, have until now remained in a condition of great vagueness and have consequently been incapable of giving a true and effective explana-tion of either of the series of phenomena which were being compared together.

Now this property of specific accumulation which

we have supposed to exist both in germinal and somatic elements, and which is the keystone of the arch in the construction of our centro-epigenetic theory, is a mnemonic faculty in the proper sense of the word. We refer, of course, to the property in virtue of which the substance contained in each of these " specifically potential " elements which is capable, when discharged, of originating a nervous current of a certain definite variety, is also the same and only substance which this current, when acting as a current of charge, can deposit. On this view the " specific potential elements " are the real mnemonic units ; they show themselves to be the substratum of all the most varied mnemonic phenomena manifested by living substance.

We must now discuss the question, whether it is justifiable to assume this property of specific accumulation in living substance ; and now two questions distinct from one another but interconnected at once arise : the first as to the existence of specific potential energies at all ; the second as to their mode of origin if they exist.

The first question is connected in several respects to that raised by Johannes Müller, and which Hering has later more fully elaborated.

The theories of Hering which, in so far as they relate to the nervous system in the strict sense he has summarised and re-stated on May 21st, 1898, in his address to the Academy of Vienna, entitled " Zur Theorie der Nerventhätigkeit," assume, rather unnecessarily, that there should be as many different paths for conducting nervous energy as there are different types of nervous energy accumulated in the different nerve centres. These theories of Müller and Hering have been later adopted and supported by Mach himself in his " Analyse der Empfindungen," and later in his last work " Erkenntnis und Irrtum," in which he assumes it to be necessary to postulate at each point of the organism, corresponding to its specific functional activity at that point—and consequently in each gland and in each muscle-cell, as well as in each element of each sense organ, and even in every point of the cerebral cortex,—a corresponding number of specific accumulations which require only to be released.

If we now admit the existence of these " specific accumulations " the second question arises, whether we can assume that they are formed and deposited by exactly the same type of specific energy as that to which they are capable of giving rise when discharged.

It seems to us that we shall be led to admit this hypothesis if we associate certain ideas most commonly accepted by biologists as to the nature of irritability in general, with certain deductions which can be drawn from the phenomena of " psychic memory " in the strict sense.

On the one hand, some biologists assume that " irritable substance " is " a system of material particles endowed with potential energy at a high degree of tension in a condition of unstable equilibrium " (Oscar Hertwig) ; and the majority agree in assuming, following in this the theories of Müller and Hertwig, combined with those of Claude Bernard, that the different types of specific activity, to which the different types of potential energy give rise, and which constitute a corresponding number of varieties of irritability of living material, are only so many specific modes of being of the same single elementary phenomenon peculiar to living matter.

On the other hand, even if we leave out of account the innumerable instances which show that the physiological effects of the mnemonic revival of sensation are the same as the effects of real sensations, we have the experiment of Wundt, in which the calling up of a vivid memory of a given colour, whilst the observer gazed fixedly at a white surface or a white figure, produced in the object gazed at the appearance of the complementary colour. This and similar experiments suggested by it, which were subsequently carried out, suffice to prove, as was affirmed by Maudsley, that the memory of a sensation is nothing but the restitution of the very same specific current which constituted the original sensation.

It follows that the specific accumulation in a given psychic sensory centre, on which its specific irritability exclusively depends, is caused by the deposit produced by the passage through this centre of the specific nervous current which this centre can now produce as " current of discharge," but which previously acted as " current of charge."

If this conclusion is irresistibly suggested with respect to the phenomena of memory in the narrower sense, where the nervous energy produced by the discharge comes into the foreground, whilst the physico-chemical phenomena accompanying it are relegated to the background, we are justified in assuming the same to be true for physiological phenomena in the stricter sense, where the physico-chemical phenomena constituting the physiological function properly so-called (muscular contraction, glandular secretion, etc.) occupy the foreground, whilst the nervous phenomena accompanying the reaction are either pushed into the background or remain totally ignored. This assumption, we may remind our readers, is in accordance with the fundamental idea of Claude Bernard as to the essentially similar nature of all irritability of organised matter, and in accordance also with the conclusion at which we have already arrived, that memory is a fundamental property of all living matter.

A third question now arises as to the nature of this specific thing which is susceptible of accumulation. Although as things stand to-day many will consider it premature to deal with this question, we cannot avoid the attempt to do so, were it only with the object of attracting to the subject the attention which it deserves.

Certain dynamic considerations, moreover, seem to justify certain vague conjectures on the subject. We must continually remind our readers that in the pages which follow we are not undertaking the exposition of a detailed hypothesis, but that we are merely advancing a few simple provisional conjectures, on the admissibility and the greater or less suggestiveness of which we are the first to feel the need of the judgment of all those who have thought of these questions.

The various forms of energy in the inorganic world

are represented, as everyone knows, as products of two factors, of which one expresses the capacity and the other the intensity or potential.

Thus the capacity factor in electrical energy is given by the quantity of electricity measured in coulombs or ampères, and the intensity factor by the potential or electro-motive force which is measured in volts. If we assume the existence of similar factors in nervous energy, may not the specific character of the various types of nervous current be in some way of the same nature as the " capacity " factor ?

If we follow up this thought, let us recall the fact that in electrical energy the capacity factor, represented by the quantity of electricity, is supposed to be made up of elements termed " electrons " all of the same capacity, no matter of what current they may be constituent parts. In mechanical energy, on the contrary, the " capacity " factor is represented by mass ; and mass is supposed to be made up of elements termed " molecular masses," which are specific for each substance—that is to say, they are of different capacity in different substances.

Now would it not be possible to imagine that the " capacity " factor of nervous energy should be also divided into elements, which, on the analogy of the electrons of currents of electricity we shall term " *nervions*," but which we shall assume to be specific for each current, and therefore of different capacity in different currents ? Further, could we not imagine that these different capacities of the specific elements were determined by as many specific varieties or

modes of action of one kind or several kinds of physico-
chemical energy which make up the stimulus exerted
both by the external and by the internal medium ?   In
other words, could we not, for instance, imagine that
the nervous current which constitutes the sensation
of red and the memory of that colour, might be made
up of a very large number of neurons all of the same
capacity, whilst another nervous current, for instance
that which constitutes the sensation of green or the
memory of that colour, might be made up of another
kind of nervions, all similarly of the same capacity,
but different from that of the nervions which make
up the nervous current giving rise to the sensation
previously mentioned ?

Let us remind ourselves that such a hypothesis
would immediately explain the universal reciprocal
correspondence between the specificity of the current
and the specificity of the deposit.   For it is easy to
picture to oneself that two molecules of different
structure would by their sudden decomposition give
rise at the same time to different products which
would represent the function or biochemical reaction
in the narrower sense, and also to energetical nervous
shocks of different capacities ;   and on the other
hand it is not inconceivable that this process might
be reversible ;   that is, that if the same energetical
nervous shock took place in the opposite direction
it might rebuild the molecular edifice which had been
broken down.   This is the more probable, as in the
case of the molecules which we are considering, it
would very probably not be a question of complete
destruction, which could only be repaired by a

reconstruction from the foundations, but perhaps merely of the separation of a given lateral group of atoms previously united to the central part of the molecule by the interposition of the imine radicle NH, or the amine radicle NH_2, or the carboxyl radicle CO.OH, or some other similar radicle. It would thus be merely a matter of reattaching the lateral group to the central mass of the molecule.

Thus Verworn, in his hypothesis of the living molecule or " biogen," imagines that in catabolism the non-nitrogenous groups of atoms are alone detached, whilst the nitrogenous groups remain and constitute the central mass of the biogen. This central mass later restores its original complexity at the expense of new non-nitrogenous groups similar to those cast off, which are contained in the surrounding nutritive medium. On the other hand we learn from organic chemistry that central molecular masses of the same composition may serve as supports for the most varied types of lateral groups or chains of atoms. If all sorts of these chains are present, ready-made in the nutritive fluid, we may well assume that *when the same amount of energy " capacity,"* which has already been produced by the detachment of a given lateral group, is again propagated through the nutritive fluid, it only sets in vibration the same quantity of mass, that is the same atomic group, selecting it along from amongst all the others which are present with it in the liquid, and thus causing its re-union with the central mass of the biogen. If further in the nutritive liquid there is present a great variety of lateral chains and of central masses of all possible kinds, we can understand how new types of energetical nervous shocks due to the impact of novel kinds of stimuli originating in the external world might give rise to quite new kinds of specific deposit which would be capable in turn of producing, by their decomposition, the same energetic nervous shocks as those which produced them.

Let us now enquire whether the properties which we have ascribed to nervous currents or discharges are capable of explaining certain characteristics presented by certain phenomena which are directly produced by nervous currents.

In order to do this we may first of all consider two extreme cases between which we can assume that every possible intermediate condition may exist. In one case we might imagine that the molecules which are capable of originating the same specific variety of discharge are arranged in groups parallel to one another, and in the second case we might suppose that they were arranged in series. In the first case the result will be a current of great capacity, but of very small potential ; in the second a current of small capacity, equal in fact to the capacity of the discharge of a single elementary accumulator, but of high potential. In this latter case the nervomotive force will be proportional to the number of molecules arranged in series, that is to say to the quantity of the specific deposit.

Ciamician, at the meeting of the Italian Society for the Advancement of Science held at Parma, in September 1907, put forward the hypothesis that in vital energy the intensity factor is represented by

" will-power." According to his view plants possess a feeble vital potential, that is will power, but a large quantity of life. Animals on the other hand are more active for the opposite reason ; amongst insects in particular, on account of their small dimensions, it is reasonable to suppose that the " capacity " factor is small, whilst the will power stands at a very high level. Since " will-power " is only nervomotive force, this is the same thing, according to our hypothesis, as saying that in organisms with strong will power (or at least in some of their tissues—nervous and muscular for instance) it is the serial type of molecular arrangement which prevails, whilst in those with a great quantity of life and feeble will power—such as we might figuratively term " phlegmatics "—it is the parallel type of arrangement of molecules which is predominant.

Let us now stop for a moment to consider the second extreme case, in which all the molecules of each specific accumulation are arranged in series, since this is the simplest case and the most interesting to us. For each parallel arrangement of molecular groups may be always considered to be constituted by as many serial accumulations arranged parallel to each other, and thus the general deductions which we may draw from the consideration of the extreme case of serial arrangement will also be applicable, with certain qualifications, to all the other types of arrangement.

In this extreme case in which all the molecules of each specific accumulation are set in series, the capacity factor will always be the same for all the discharges, because it will always be equal to the capacity of discharge of a single molecule. In other words, this capacity factor for all the discharges to which this specific accumulation can give rise, will be a constant, independent of all the other circumstances which may be present at the moment of discharge. This specific accumulation therefore will either not discharge itself at all, or, if it discharges itself, will always give the same capacity of current, that is, the capacity of a single one of its " nervions."

We may then enquire whether it is just because the capacity of discharge for each specific accumulation cannot vary, that the accumulation is in most cases only discharged—or as we say " released "—when the same currents or a portion of the same currents are active in its neighbourhood, which were active when it was deposited for the first time. Because only when this is so, will the alteration which the discharge of such a fixed capacity will produce in the neighbouring circulation of nervous currents, be reduced to a minimum and will consequently require for its production a very limited amount of nervo-motive force. Something analogous would be produced in an arrangement of several electric accumulators in the same circuit if each one of them could give rise only to a current of a certain fixed intensity, different for each accumulator—the accumulator, the particular intensity of whose discharge would produce a notable alteration in the distribution of electrical energy in the circuit, will be prevented or " inhibited " from discharging itself unless its electro-motive force is high enough to overcome the resistance of the other currents of the circuit to its discharge.

The phenomena of the association or succession of ideas and generally all forms of psychical or physiological association, which constitute the keystone of the arch and the foundation stone, not only of psychology, but of all biology, as well as the opposite phenomena of psycho-physiological inhibition, might thus be the direct consequences of the constancy of the " capacity " of discharge exhibited by each of the different specific accumulations.

Thus we could explain—as we may here mention in parenthesis—why the " specific potential elements " of the germ-plasm can become active only when the embryo has reached the ontogenetic stage corresponding to the phylogenetic stage immediately preceding that in which this particular " specific potential element " was deposited for the first time in the germ-plasm.

We may remark on the subject of the association of ideas that the difficulty is not so much to understand why certain ideas recall certain other ideas, but why certain ideas recall *only* certain others. For if we consider the enormous number of nervous connections which connect all the psychic centres with one another —a number which in the human brain, according to the calculations of Fleschig, would amount to several millions, and which if placed end to end would attain a length of thousands of kilometres—we should naturally expect that the stimulation of a single psychic centre would affect all the others and would produce an extremely irregular and chaotic association of ideas.

It was just in order to explain this " limitation of

association " that Hering, as we have seen above, invented the theory, not only of the specific nature of the accumulations of energy in different centres, but also of the specific character of the paths connecting the centres with each other ; for this reason also the supporters of the neurone theory have put forward the idea of raising of " drawbridges " connecting the neurones, that is of the retraction of the majority of the dendritic processes of the neurone as a consequence of which it would be isolated from all the other neurones—except those from which it is arranged that it shall receive stimulation. But Hering's theory leads to the consequence that the association of ideas should be fixed and stereotyped ; and with this conclusion the most familiar facts of mnemonic recollection and imagination and even of dreams are totally irreconcileable. The other hypothesis, viz., that of drawbridges, does not exhaust the problem, for it does not tell us why the neurone lifts certain drawbridges and leaves others down. Besides, this neurone theory will probably soon be replaced by the theory that there is always an effective anatomical continuity of the entire nervous system.

If such a continuity exists, and if we consider how close a network connects the different nervous elements with one another and the impossibility of assuming that the different strands in this network have each its " specific character," so that each can conduct only one specific variety of current, we shall have reason to suspect that the causes of the reciprocal and limited " release " of certain nervous currents by others must be sought in the " energetic " properties of the currents themselves and in their dynamic relations to one another.

But we must content ourselves here with this brief sketch, in order to allude equally to other interconnected questions, viz., those respecting the nature of assimilation and the trophic effect exerted by functional activity and the rejuvenation produced by fertilisation. We must, however, again emphasise the fact that the hypothesis which we are about to put forward must be regarded as purely provisional, and its acceptance or rejection in no way involves the legitimacy of the other hypothesis, viz., that of specific accumulations, for although the latter hypothesis suggests and supports the hypothesis which we are now putting forward, it is really quite independent of it.

What, above all, strikes the biologist about assimilation is that it is not a process of continual production, but of continual *reproduction* since it incessantly reproduces organic substance in proportion as this is consumed. "One might say," writes Oscar Hertwig, "that life is only an incessant process of destruction and renewed formation of organic substance." Such a process indeed exhibits all the characters of a true mnemonic phenomenon. As a matter of fact every specific substance which consumes itself in giving rise to its proper functional activity, restores itself whatever (within certain limits) may be the nature of its nutritive medium, so as to remain always "specifically identical to itself," just as if it was formed and deposited by its own specific activity which being at first destructive, then becomes constructive. We are led to suppose that assimilation is at bottom a duplex phenomenon, viz., the excitement of the specific activity and then the deposition by this of its own specific deposit.

Quite independently of these considerations other fundamental vital phenomena have led biologists to conclusions in accordance with this supposition. Such are the facts of fertilisation and of conjugation in general, which may be reduced to a simple " coupling " of the chromosomes of the male nucleus with those of the female nucleus; the reducing or " meiotic " division with which the process of maturation concludes in both types of germ-cells, by which the normal number of chromosomes of the egg is halved in order to make room for the reception of the chromosomes of the fertilizing nucleus, which have likewise been reduced to half the normal number; the strange nuclear process of synapsis with which maturation begins both in the ovum and in the spermatozoon, which brings to view extremely delicate threads like necklaces arranged in pairs parallel to one another, so that each minute grain of one filament is opposed to a similar grain of the other filament; the coupling of granules of chromatin in many other nuclear phases, both of germinal and of somatic cells; the constant appearance in couples of all the microscopic elements of nuclei between which, we have strong reason to suspect, take place the production of vital phenomena. All these phenomena have already suggested to more than one biologist the idea that vital energy can neither be produced nor maintained, except between couples of material elements of opposite character acting, as in the absence of a precise hypothesis it has been vaguely expressed, in the manner of " opposite poles."

At the same time the complete qualitative equivalence of the chromosomes of the two sexes, an equivalence which can be indirectly deduced from their capacity of transmitting the same hereditary qualities, and directly proved by certain interesting experiments of the substitution of the nucleus of a spermatozoon for the nucleus of an egg, and by the self-fertilisation of the nucleus of an egg after the reducing division by the nucleus of the polar body, leads us to believe that the opposed members of these elementary couples are qualitatively equal to one another.

We might then risk the suggestion that the alleged " opposite poles," which together constitute the vital element, are nothing at bottom but two sets of serially arranged accumulators, specifically equal to one another, but of different potentials, and placed opposite to one another, between which an oscillating nervous discharge is produced similar in certain respects to the oscillating electrical discharges of the resonators of Hertz. Perhaps we might regard the reinforcement of these latter oscillations by synchronous Hertzian waves and the reinforcement of the oscillating intra-nuclear discharges of nervous energy by synchronous oscillations of light and heat as the same phenomenon, for the heat and light rays are themselves Hertzian waves, albeit infinitely short ones. On this point a fact recorded by Engelmann is most interesting ; he observed that those colours in the spectrum which are most readily absorbed by bacteria are those which are most favourable to their metabolism. *This metabolism would thus appear to be a phenomenon of a vibratory nature capable of undergoing resonance.*

We should obtain in this manner an automatic process of the growth of the nuclear substance which would, however, be slowed down and eventually stopped by the progressive equalisation of the " nervo-motive " force in the two opposite and coupled accumulators.

From this we could deduce the trophic action exerted by every process which is capable of re-establishing a state of inequality between the opposed " nervo-motive " forces and, consequently, the trophic action exerted by every extra-nuclear functional discharge of one or other of the two accumulators which would reduce the nervo-motive force of the accumulator thus discharged. This is in accordance with the observation of Claude Bernard that " the phenomena of functional destruction are themselves the precursors and instigators of that organic restitution which takes place during the so-called periods of functional repose."

From the same principle we could also deduce the explanation of the rejuvenating influence exerted by fertilisation or by conjugation which on this view would consist in substituting in each mnemonic element of the germ-plasm for one of the two accumulators, which had a " nervo-motive " force equal to that of its fellow, another accumulator specifically identical, but endowed with an amount of " nervo-motive " force quantitatively different. Fertilisation or conjugation has been regarded by most biologists since Spencer's time as equivalent to the disturbance of an equilibrium which rendered the maintenance of vital activity impossible, whence the possibility of replacing this fertilisation or conjugation by renewed functional activity or any other kind of disturbance as the experiments of Maupas have shown to be the case in Infusoria.

We might also ultimately deduce the universal tendency of life under the influence of thermic energy to expand indefinitely, that is, as Mach has expressed it, " to draw within its own sphere even larger quantities of matter "—a tendency which has impelled many biologists, and Ostwald in particular, to compare life to fire.

We have now completed the description of the energetic properties which we have supposed to characterise nervous energy, that base of all life. We are the first to admit, as we think it necessary to repeat once again, that the hypotheses which we have put forward are nothing more at most than a first quite provisional attempt at a solution and one which is sketched only in baldest outlines. They have been put forward with the sole aim of directing the attention of biologists and " natural philosophers " to these problems, and of arousing on the part of specialists of very diverse branches of science the most searching critical examination of our views, which alone will separate the more firmly based from the baseless parts of our hypotheses.

We admit that in postulating the properties with which we have endowed nervous energy we have introduced a form of energy which at present we cannot reduce to any of the other forms of physico-chemical energy so far known. In a word, we have imagined such a form of energy, which, though of course subject to the general laws of energetics, would nevertheless differ by the possession of certain well-defined fundamental qualities from all the other forms of energy in the same way as these differ from one another. But no " natural philosopher," no " energetist," and not even a physicist who does not take too narrow and limited view of natural phenomena would be prepared to assert that such an assumption would conflict with the more solid results which science has so far achieved.

CHAPTER V

THE MNEMONIC THEORY OF SEMON

Terminology of Semon. Engraphic action and ecphoric stimuli. The property of organic material of being subject to engraphic influence may be regarded as a preservative principle. Engrams acquired during the life of the individual and engraphic tendencies to irritability not acquired during the life of the individual : the experiment of Claypole on just hatched ostriches, behaviour of a young magpie in presence of a dish full of water, the removal of a caterpillar from one cocoon to another in a different stage of formation, behaviour of young birds placed in an artificial nest. All ontogenetic phenomena are also capable of being included in the category of inborn engraphic tendencies to irritability. The deficiencies in Semon's theory : his rejection of the idea of mnemonic localisation and the absence of any hypothesis as to the nature of mnemonic action. Like previous mnemonic theories Semon's theory still remains indefinite.

AFTER having in the previous chapters expounded in all its details our centro-epigenetic hypothesis, which is indeed also a mnemonic theory of development, it would seem to be profitable for purposes of comparison to give a rapid analysis of the fundamental contents of Semon's theory as set forth in his work " Die Mneme als erhaltendes Prinzip im Wechsel des organischen Geschehens." In this publication he has taken up and developed further the attractive idea which Hering advanced as long ago as 1870 in his celebrated address to the Academy of Vienna which was entitled " Ueber das Gedächtnis als eine allgemeine Funktion der organischen Materie." Since Semon's theory is at once a synthesis and

the most perfect development of all preceding
mnemonic theories it is of great importance that it
should be compared with our theory.

Semon's begins by giving definitions of the terms in
the new terminology which he has adopted. He calls
the condition of living substance before a given
stimulus reaches it " the primary indifferent state,"
and its condition after the stimulus, " the secondary
indifferent state." " Whatever may be the kingdom
to which the organism belongs," he goes on to say,
" whether it be a protist, an animal or a plant it is
easy to show in a number of cases that when an
organism, after the cessation of a stimulus, has
attained the secondary indifferent state, it has undergone a permanent change. I call this effect of
stimuli, ' engraphic action,' because it is, so to speak,
carved in or impressed on the living substance ; to
each change of the living substance I give the name
of the ' engram ' of the stimulus which produces it,
and I term ' mneme ' the whole number of the
engrams which this organism has inherited or
acquired during its individual life ; from this follows
immediately the distinction between an inherited
' mneme,' and one which has been acquired by the
individual. I call ' mnemonic phenomena ' those
phenomena exhibited by an organism which are the
result of a given engram or of a number of these
engrams."

The result of engraphic action, in consequence of the
permanent change which it produces in living matter,
is that the state of excitement which a given stimulus
has produced in the past may be reproduced, not only

by a repetition of the same stimulus, but also by other influences to which on this account Semon has given the name of " ecphoric stimuli " or " ecphoric influences." Thus for instance if the stimulus a when it first occurs produces the reaction A and the stimulus b only the reaction B, the reaction $(A+B)$ when it occurs for the first time can only be called forth by the stimulus $(a+b)$. But when this same reaction $(A+B)$ is evoked as a mnemomic response, that is as an effect of the engram produced by a former stimulus $(a+b)$, then this response can be called forth by the stimulus a alone, or by the stimulus b alone, either of these stimuli now acting as an " ecphoric " stimulus.

In the same way a stimulus which, if it acted for the first time, would be too weak to produce a reaction, when it acts as " ecphoric stimulus " may be more than sufficient to evoke a response of such an amount as it could have produced as original stimulus only if it had been of considerably greater intensity.

This power of living substance, not only of being excited by a stimulus but of retaining engraphic impressions so that it is able to return to the same complex state of excitation as a result of a very feeble or of a very partial repetition of the same stimulus as had produced this state in the first instance, may be regarded as a conservative factor (*als erhaltendes Prinzip*) in the continual changes undergone by this substance under the influences of stimulation raining in upon it from the outer world, a stimulation which is continually varying in character and which never occurs twice in absolutely the same manner.

BIOLOGICAL MEMORY

After having discussed the mnemonic phenomena produced by the engrams acquired during the life of the individual, Semon goes on to consider quite a different series of phenomena which lead him to the following conclusion : " In the irritable material of protists, animals and plants, we find properties termed ' irritable dispositions ' (certainly not acquired during the life-time of the individual) which, as is denoted by this very term ' dispositions,' are usually latent. But certain definite influences can activate them or ' release ' them from this latent condition, just as happens to the engrams acquired by the individual, after which they become latent again. Each repetition of the ecphoric influence evokes again the corresponding state of irritation which manifests itself by its appropriate reaction."

It is in the suggestive description of this series of phenomena, made in such a way as to indicate the conclusion just alluded to as their only adequate explanation, that the great merit and chief originality of Semon's work consists. Amongst the various cases referred to by that author we shall only allude to a few which we have chosen as the most typical and which are as follows :

According to Claypole, newly-hatched ostriches in the artificial incubator only begin to peck at their food when someone strikes with a stick or similar object in front of them on the ground where the corn is scattered. " Of all explanations of this fact," adds Semon, " that which appears most probable is that which attributes it to the ' ecphory ' of an inherited engram, and to be precise an engram of which the corresponding reaction is the act of pecking; in this case the ecphoric stimulus is the reproduction of the original stimulus a little altered; that is to say that the educative influence of the act of pecking carried out by the mother in the presence of her young is replaced by that of striking gently on the food with the finger nail or another pointed object."

The next instance is still more typical. In the cage of a young magpie, about five weeks old, which he had reared from the egg, the observer placed a dish of water. The bird pecked twice at the water, after which, although it had never previously been in the water, and although it remained all the time outside the dish, it began to make all the movements usually carried out by a bird when it bathes itself : it drew back its head, shook itself and moved its wings and its tail and finally strutted proudly around. " This case also," adds our author, " loses its astonishing character if we assume that we are dealing with an inherited engram on which the stimulus of contact with the water acts ecphorically, although this stimulus affects only a small portion of the body."

Huber relates the case of a caterpillar which by a series of actions manufactures for the purposes of its pupation a very complicated web. Now he found that if he placed one of these caterpillars which had arrived at the sixth stage of its work on another web which was only completed as far as the third stage, far from evidencing the slightest embarrassment it repeated perfectly the fourth, fifth and sixth stages of the construction of the web. On the other hand, if he took a caterpillar from a web in the third stage and

placed it in another web which had been completed
as far as the ninth stage so that the insect would be in a
position to spare itself the greater part of its labour,
then the caterpillar was utterly unable to omit the
intermediate stages and to begin its work at the ninth
stage ; it began work at the third stage which it had
just left unfinished, so that in the new web which the
creature proceeded to spin the fourth, fifth, sixth,
seventh and eighth stages were spun twice. These
facts are interpreted by Semon in the following
manner. " The caterpillar is in a similar condition
to that in which we find ourselves when we have to
recite a piece of poetry which we have often recited
before. We can easily repeat it from the beginning
to the end, but we are not in a position to begin it and
carry it on starting from any given point on the mere
suggestion of a whispered word. At least, we are not
able to do it at the first attempt. If, however, we have
recited, even if only once, a given portion in a loud
voice, then we can within the limits of this portion
commence and repeat any part of it starting from any
point whatsoever."

We know that birds brought up in an incubator
which have never in their lives seen a nest, begin at
once to build a nest when the opportunity to mate is
afforded them, and that they succeed in building nests
quite similar to, if not so perfect, as those built by
other adults which have built nests before, these latter
adults having presumably learnt to build nests through
seeing them built by older and more experienced birds.
Now this impulse to build a nest can be suppressed by
presenting to the birds a completed nest, provided

that it does not differ too much from the nest peculiar to the species.

The most remarkable fact in connection with this nest-building instinct is that if the nest shown to the bird while not so different from the typical nest as to be rejected is, nevertheless, obviously dissimilar to this, the bird will set about correcting it by throwing away what is abnormal in it and replacing what is wanting. We have to remember that this is done by birds which in their individual lives have never seen a nest and which have no personal experience of egg-laying or of the young which they are going to produce for the first time. " The characteristic feature of these processes," Semon justly goes on to say, " is that the normal succession of reactions is modified by the actual complex stimulus exerted by the nest offered to the birds in such a way that it corresponds to the difference between this actual stimulus and the ultimate effect of the mnemonic excitation which would have consisted in the construction of the typical nest of the species. In other words, in so far as the actual complex stimulus exerted on the animal by the nest offered to it exhibits divergencies from the stimulus which would have been normally produced by the nest built in consequence of mnemonic reactions, it calls forth different reactions on the part of the animals in order to remove these divergencies. Now this impulse to remove the difference between an actual complex impression and the similar impression called up by the memory is one of the most characteristic manifestations of mnemonic activity. Therefore, regarded in this light, the inborn instinct to construct a nest is seen to be a mnemonic pheno-menon."

After having thus shown that many " tendencies to irritability " of organisms which have certainly not been acquired during their individual lives, neverthe-less behave exactly like engrams acquired during life, if we may judge from their modes of excitation and of manifestation, Semon goes on to point out that not merely the cases of development which we have just described which might almost be said to be of a psychic character, but all ontogenetic phenomena, including those which might be termed morphogenetic in the narrower sense, can be comprised within the category of engraphic " tendencies to irritability."

His proof of this proposition is especially based on the fact that the morphological passage from one stage of development to another is evoked by stimuli which, on account of their nature, or of the conditions of the environment within which they work, could certainly never exert a true " formative " action ; but which may be easily interpreted as " ecphoric stimuli " acting on an engram or on a given series of engrams which the species has acquired during its past history, as, for instance, when certain amphibia, in order to begin their metamorphosis from gilled animals to pulmonate animals, require previously to come into contact with atmospheric air.

If this explanation is valid, that is to say, if the phenomena of normal development are also to be attributed to the " ecphoric release " of one or of a series of engrams, it follows that many of the special morphogenetic phenomena are susceptible of a new explanation fundamentally similar to that given of phenomena belonging to a purely psychic category. Thus, to give one instance, the tendency of organisms to restore their normal form when this has been destroyed, as happens when an amputated member is regenerated, would be nothing but the tendency to do away with the divergencies between the actual abnormal morphological condition and the normal morphological condition mnemonically recalled. This tendency would consequently be of the same essential character as that described above, manifested by the bird which begins to alter the nest presented to it, until this nest has been made to conform to the type peculiar to the species.

Such is a brief and impartial summary of the theory of Semon. However attractively and masterfully it has been expounded by him we feel bound to add a word on a fundamental difficulty which Semon has necessarily encountered in his exposition of it, and which we do not think that he has successfully surmounted.

Since the facts force us to assume that some of the most characteristic engrams acquired during life, as for instance ordinary memories, must be localised in certain parts of the body, Semon is much embarassed in trying to explain how these engrams are transmitted in heredity, since their position has no relation to that of the germ-cells by means of which they must nevertheless be transmitted.

His attempt to escape from this dilemma consists in its essence of a denial, in defiance of facts, that there is a real localisation even of ordinary memories. He substitutes for localisation a hypothetical diffusion of each engraphic effect, psychical as well as morpho-genetic, whether simple or complex, and therefore of each engram. This diffusion he pictures as spreading out from the limited zone where the action is at its maximum intensity and reaching with continually decreasing intensity, but without alteration of quality, not only all the cells of the body including the germ cells, but even each of the smallest living units of each cell to which Semon gives the name " protomeres."

Now we need not emphasise the objection that, as we have already stated, such an assumption is in direct contradiction with the best ascertained facts, such as those which are provided by diseases of memory in which we can demonstrate that there is a true localisation of mnemonic phenomena because each category of impressions of which the memory is lost is always correlated with a definite lesion of a well-defined region of the brain or the rest of the nervous system. We need only ask what intelligible meaning could we attach to this diffusion of each engraphic action, psychic or morphogenetic, even of the utmost complexity, which is supposed to take place in such a way that the effect remains qualitatively the same though of differing degrees of intensity throughout all the minutest constituents of the organism, as for instance the diffusion of a visual impression to mus-cular fibres, glandular cells and so forth, or the diffusion of a local functional adaptation throughout the entire organism? What, indeed, but a purely verbal explanation, devoid of anything comparable with any phenomenon or model known to us, is gained by suggesting that the inheritability of the innumerable engrams which make up the entire ontogeny, both those acquired during the life of the indvidual and those inherited, of both psychic and morphogenetic type, is due to the accumulation of all these engrams in each " protomere " of the germ-plasm ?

Semon's theory, therefore, suffers the fate of all the similar mnemonic theories of heredity which have preceded it. This is indeed inevitable, because the close comparison of the phenomena of memory in the narrow sense with ontogenetic phenomena, though many have recognised that this comparison enshrines a fundamental truth, will be unable to yield any positive results so long as we decline to put forward any hypothesis as to the nature of mnemonic property, and so long as we do not recognise the existence of a true localisation of the morphogenetic memory of the species, such as exists for the psychic memory acquired by the individual during his life.

As the reader has learnt from the previous chapters, in which a short account only of this subject is given, it is just these two points which we have dealt with in our work entitled " On the Inheritance of Acquired Characters," which have led us to advance the hypotheses of specific accumulation and of centro-epigenesis, which seem to us to give a perfectly satisfactory explanation of the mechanism of this " transmission of engrams."

It is for this reason that, in concluding what we have to say on the work of Semon, we find ourselves in a position to give the following impartial answer to the question which he himself has raised, viz., whether by his new terminology he has done anything beyond expressing in other words the facts he has endeavoured to explain. We find that the result of his studies is something very far indeed from being a mere different mode of the expression of well-known facts. His new nomenclature, his careful choice of facts, and his ingenious method of arranging them and of discussing them, has succeeded in impressing on the scientific mind, in a much more suggestive manner than any of his predecessors, the idea that the instincts and the other inborn tendencies of the organism, including the morphogenetic tendencies, on account of the circumstances in which they become active and of the nature of their manifestations, are very probably nothing but " engrams " which the ancestors of the particular individual have acquired during their lives and which they have transmitted to the particular individual by heredity. This statement of the result which he has obtained is sufficient to make us appreciate the worth and importance of his work. But he has not succeeded in throwing the least light on the nature of this engraphic action nor on the way in which the engrams are transmitted from father to son, and this circumstance does much to discredit his theory, for it is on this account that he does not succeed in removing from his affirmation of the identity of mnemonic phenomena in the narrower sense and morphogenetic processes, the appearance of being a forced comparison with one another of phenomena of essentially different nature.

CHAPTER VI

A Botanical Supporter of Mnemonic Theories

Sir Francis Darwin as a decided partisan of mnemonic theories. He, too, assumes that the system of protoplasmic bridges forms an "idioplasmic" network penetrating the smallest recesses of the organism. He, however, refuses to assume, as Semon is obliged to do, that every local change, whilst remaining qualitatively the same, is propagated throughout the entire organism. He accepts as an alternative to Semon's view our centro-epigenetic theory which solves this difficulty of mnemonic localisation. He demonstrates the essential identity throughout the vegetable kingdom of the temporary variations of form, that is the movements, and of the permanent variations of form or morphological changes. By the demonstration of this identity, Darwin makes a contribution of the greatest importance to the confirmation of our centro-epigenetic theory.

OUR centro-epigenetic hypothesis expounded in the second and third chapters of this work and Semon's theory of which we have given an abstract in the preceding chapter, are founded principally, although not exclusively, on the facts observed in the animal kingdom. It appears, therefore, to be a matter of great importance in the confirmation of mnemonic theories in general and of our centro-epigenetic theory in particular, that a botanist of the reputation of Sir Francis Darwin should support them, a botanist, who, by his remarkable studies on the life, movements and sensations of plants has worthily continued the traditions of his illustrious father.

Sir Francis Darwin, who delivered the Presidential Address to the British Association for the Advancement of Science in 1908, on the occasion of the annual meeting of the Association held in Dublin, reminded his hearers that that year was the 50th anniversary of the publication of the two works by Charles Darwin and Alfred Wallace on the origin of species. After he had reviewed in masterly fashion some of the most hotly debated questions relating to the development of organisms, he declared himself to be a decided adherent of the mnemonic theories. Nevertheless, with great impartiality, whilst emphasising the light which these theories threw on the phenomena of development, and showing on what a series of well attested observations they were based, he did not omit to mention their weak point, which results from the difficult question which is raised by them concerning the mode of the hereditary transmission.

This question is concerned with the way in which morphological changes, produced in the body by its continual adaptation to the successive changes in the environment, could leave mnemonic traces of themselves in the nuclei of the germ-cells. Of course, it is not the mere fact of transmission in itself which seems inconceivable. As Sir Francis Darwin himself has recognised, the system of intercellular protoplasmic bridges supplies us, even in cases such as those of the plants where the nervous system with all its fibres and fibrillæ is wanting, with that idioplasmic network penetrating all the recesses of the organism which Nägeli dreamed of. This network, Nägeli imagined, would allow every local disturbance of the body to diffuse its echo throughout all the other parts of the body, including the germ cells.

What is difficult to imagine is, how a local morphological change, produced by the environment in any given part of the body, even when this change is not uniform at all points, could, as Semon supposed, be resolved into and propagated through the rest of the body as an impulse or excitation of a definite kind, which, whilst diminishing in intensity, would nevertheless remain qualitatively identical with itself, until it imprinted itself on the nuclei of the germ cells where it was preserved so as to be capable at a given moment of being restored or evoked. A further difficulty was to conceive how the diffusion of this particular impulse, proceeding from a given part of the body, could remain distinct from and independent of other similar impulses produced at the same time by the most varied local changes in all the other parts of the body.

Sir Francis Darwin suggested, therefore, our centro-epigenetic theory as an alternative to Semon's hypothesis, which has some analogy with Charles Darwin's theory of pangenesis. Semon, in fact, has merely substituted for Darwin's " pangenes," which were supposed to be produced in all the cells of the body by the changes in the environment, and which differed from cell to cell, the transmission by nervous paths of all the new impressions or local engrams, differing from point to point of the organism, produced by every new external stimulus.

Sir Francis Darwin supported the centro-epigenetic theory just because according to it the

" excitation " does not remain unchanged as it passes
from one point to another of the organism. On the
contrary, as it traverses each nucleus it changes its
character either as a result of the direct modifying
action exercised on it by that nucleus or of its combination with all the other " excitations " or impulses
which at that instant converge to meet in that nucleus.
It follows that at each point of the organism, and
consequently also in the point where the germinal
substance is situated, there will be at one and the
same time only a single resultant excitation whose
specific nature, though variable from point to point,
will be the function and expression of the general state
of the nervous circulation made up of all the nervous
impulses passing through the body which constitute,
taken together, the complex physiologico-morphological state of the organism.

The successive physiologico-morphological states
which make up the successive phylogenetic stages
traversed by a given species, will each produce in the
germinal substance, which is always situated in the
same relative position in the organism, a corresponding
resultant excitation, and each such resultant excitation will in its turn leave in the germ-plasm a mnemonic
impression or accumulation capable of restoring in
each new ontogeny the same specific " excitation "
which gave rise to it. It is sufficient then to assume
that the germinal substance is always situated in the
same place, both when it is receiving and accumulating
resultant impressions, or when it is re-emitting them
in each new ontogeny, to explain why the developing
organism passes through all the physiologico-morpho-

logical states traversed by the species in its evolution, though, of course, this restoration of previous states may be more or less abridged ("recapitulated") according to the degree of preservation of the corresponding mnemonic deposits. In a similar way it suffices that a single point of the membrane of a phonograph should again pass through all the conditions through which it passed when the membrane received the sonorous impressions, in order that the entire membrane should again pass through all the extremely complex conditions which were originally produced in it by the external world and which are now reproduced by the action of a single internal point.

Sir Francis Darwin shows what a simplification results from our hypothesis ; for whilst, according to Weismann, as well as to Semon, the most minute particularities of structure and even the most microscopic portions of the cells of each stage in development, including the adult stage, must each be represented in the germ-plasm by a corresponding "determinant" or "engram," according to our theory, a single mnemonic element in the germinal substance is sufficient to represent and determine in its entirety the mode of being complex of each corresponding stage of the ontogeny.

But Sir Francis Darwin has made a personal contribution, and one of the highest interest, to the facts which support mnemonic theories in general and ours in particular. It is the affirmation amply developed and demonstrated by him, especially for plants, of the fundamental identity between the temporary variations of form, constituting the movements of organisms, and the definite changes of form, or morphological modifications of organisms.

If we assume this identity, and if we at the same time admit the mnemonic nature of the reproduction of movements which were previously caused by external stimuli, we should naturally deduce a similar nature for the reproduction in the plant of morphological changes. Thus, for instance, plants which sleep, bend down and subsequently re-elevate their leaves or change in some other manner the usual aspect of the leaves, according to a rhythm originally produced by the succession of day and night, as is proved by the fact that the period of this rhythm may be altered by a quicker or slower alternation of artificial light and darkness. These rhythms, whether natural or artificially modified, persist even if the plant is kept for some days in complete darkness. This persistence is obviously due to some process of mnemonic nature. Now the same thing can be seen in certain permanent morphological changes. Thus a beech tree can produce leaves of such different types that they seem to belong to two different species, according as it grows in sunlight or in shade. The ontogeny is different in the two cases, and this difference is due to a different action of the environment. But the interesting point is that there are other plants which grow best in the shade in which the shape of the leaves is similar to that of the leaves which the beech puts forth in the shade, but in which this shape has now become a permanent characteristic of the species and does not vary, whatever may be the degree of illumination to which the plant is exposed. Consequently the shape of the leaves which in the beech is determined by the environment, is produced in these plants in a purely mnemonic manner. Goebel has drawn attention to the fact that in certain orchids the assimilatory roots take on a flattened form when they are exposed to sunlight, whilst in other species this modification has become spontaneous and is manifested even when the roots are in darkness.

We may remark, moreover, that the sudden variations in form which constitute the movements of plants, whether they are caused by stimuli from the environment or whether they are produced in a mnemonic way, are effected, just as in animals, by the transmission of " excitations " or nervous impulses which pass from certain parts of the plant to other parts. Hence—and it is in this point that the theory of Sir Francis Darwin furnishes a powerful support to our centro-epigenetic hypothesis—*we must attribute to these nervous impulses, not only the movements of plants, but also their definite variation in form or morphological modifications, since we have seen that these latter are of the same nature as the movements.*

We can now see why botanists have given a much more cordial welcome to mnemonic theories than zoologists themselves. There is, in fact, in the case of the plant, a much closer dependence than in the animal of the series of morphological changes constituting development on the environment. At the same time, the movements of plants are much slower than those of animals, and they often take the form of a passage of the plant from one form to another in which it persists for a considerable time. These circumstances have rendered it easy to perceive the close analogy between morphological modifications and movements.

Moreover, the fact that plants, although completely devoid of a nervous system, manifest the phenomena of irritability, of transmission of stimuli and of memory, has lent support to the view that all the somatic nuclei are essentially similar in nature to those of the nerve centres, and that the intercellular bridges have the same power of transmitting stimuli which is possessed by the nerve fibres. Consequently it ceases to be incomprehensible that in the embryo animal during its earliest stages of development, even when it as yet possesses no nervous system, the successive phases of ontogeny could be caused by the discharge and transmission of nervous energy.

CHAPTER VII

TELEOLOGY AND MEMORY

Auguste Pauly the most orthodox representative of the new " pan-animist " theories of life. The pursuit of an end or " purposefulness " (Zweckmässigkeit) as a general property of organisms. Each new phylogenetic modification consists in the employment of already formed morphological structures to serve a new purpose. This new use is indeed a discovery or " invention " made by the animal, and this use slowly modifies the structure of the old organ. By the hypothesis that all actions now involuntary and even purely physiological actions have been in the past voluntary actions, Pauly seeks to extend indefinitely the applicability of the principle of the " auto-plasmatic " action of animals. Consequently he lapses into pan-animistic mysticism. This revival of animistic theories is caused by the inadequacy of purely physico-chemical theories. It is not the mere " adaptation " of life to actual external conditions, but the " adaptation " in anticipation to future external conditions which constitutes the exclusively peculiar property of life, and this anticipation *can only be explained by mnemonic theories.*

AFTER having in the previous chapters set forth our mnemonic theory of development and having compared it with the theory of Semon and having examined the important support for it derived from the researches of Sir Francis Darwin on the movement of plants, we must now pass to the consideration of the other fundamental characteristics of life which can be explained by our hypothesis of the nature of the mnemonic property of living substance. In the present chapter we shall compare the explanations of the purposefulness of life which are provided by the metaphysical theories, which we may term " pan-animist," of which Pauly is the best known exponent, and by our mnemonic theory. Subsequently, in the two following chapters we shall deal directly with the question of the purposefulness in all its manifestations and with the question of its essentially mnemonic character.

In his much discussed book entitled " Darwinismus und Lamarckismus, Entwurf einer psychophysischen Teleologie" (Munich, 1905), August Pauly expounds in the clearest way the fundamental difference between the Darwinian and the Lamarckian conceptions of evolution.

Darwinism, he says, in alleging that it is possible to explain all organic evolution by the struggle for existence and natural selection, regards the faculty of self-adaptation of living beings itself as a result of the accumulation of fortuitous variations, whilst on the contrary this faculty is evidently a primordial and fundamental property of life. In consequence, Darwin has continually revolved round the question without solving it and has thus done more thaȟ anyone else to prevent our obtaining a deeper and more intimate knowledge of vital phenomena. On the contrary, Lamarck attacked the problem directly and directed his attention from the first to definite instances of adaptation to an end which were correlated with changes or intensifications of functions and which consequently represented new adaptations in the act of appearing. Consequently, according to Darwin, the organism acquired all its properties in a passive manner, whereas, according to Lamarck, the organism acquired them by directly forming them for itself by its own activity.

TELEOLOGY AND MEMORY

After having thus defined the relations sustained to one another by the fundamental conceptions of Darwinism and Lamarckism respectively, Pauly, who is a supporter of Lamarck, proceeds to the study of the basal property of organisms, viz., adaptability to ends or " Zweckmässigkeit."

Every action, he observes, is purposeful, and its direction toward an end is caused by the mnemonic recollection and association of two experiences, viz., one of felt need and one of the means by which this need has previously been satisfied. This association produces a " judgment " of a psychical nature, but evidently associated in its activity with physical energy, as to the capacity of the means to satisfy the given need.

Pauly goes on to say that we learn from the study of phylogenetic history that in accomplishing each new adaptation the animal always employs as instruments those which it chances to possess, viz., already formed morphological structures which until then had served other ends, but which at a given moment the animal discovers that it can put to a new use, and that it is in consequence of the new use that these structures become slowly modified. A good instance of such modification is provided by the limbs of Crustacea which have been transformed in accordance with the use made of them by the animal, but which were originally all similar to one another.

The use for a new and completely different purpose of an instrument until then employed for another definite end, is really a true invention on the part of the animal. Some of these " inventions " have only produced results of limited importance, but others have led to results of far-reaching importance which naturally could never have been foreseen at their first origin. " We need only think," remarks Pauly, " of the importance of the results in the evolution of the human jaws and face, which flowed from the discovery that the branchial arches could be used to seize nourishment."

It is clear that each " invention " may, and in most cases will, be succeeded by another similar one which will employ for a different end what its predecessor has " invented," which in turn was produced by the modification of a still older structure, and so proceeding from invention to invention, the organism will be able to build itself up directly by its own work.

We consider that this " auto-plasmation " ought to be recognised, possibly to a much greater degree than it has been in the past, and it is the merit of Pauly to have forced it on our attention.

To maintain that in virtue of its own efforts an animal succeeds in satisfying its new needs by the use of old means, and by this new use, ever better guided by the accumulated experience of its former efforts, it changes its organs by making them constantly better adapted to the new uses—this is perhaps only to assert what has already been said about the formation of an organ by its function—but in this manner more prominence is given to the part which the intelligence of the animal is supposed to play in this modification.

This " auto-plasmation " can only be true for organs, the functions of which are controlled by the will. Let us, however, note that many acts now involuntary began as voluntary action, and it follows that the range of this auto-plasmatic action will be very greatly extended. But how far ought it to be extended ? That, indeed, is a difficult question.

The evolution of the middle finger of the hand of *Chiromys madagascariensis,* which is much longer and slenderer than the other fingers and which is employed by the animal to extract from the tubular cavities of plants the pith or insect larvæ, may have been caused by the ever-increasing skill on the part of the animal in employing this organ for this use, a skill acquired as a result of many more or less successful efforts. This will seem more probable if we assume that the contraction of the epidermis tends to make the finger more slender, and if the elongation of the muscular fibres which involves the lengthening of the bones has been, to even a small extent, under the control of the will. We might, perhaps, make the same assumptions—at any rate in part—about the formation of the great claws and other appendages of the Crustacea mentioned above, about the formation of some organs or parts of organs employed by insects for cleaning their antennæ, about the elongation of the neck and fore-limbs of the giraffe, about the legs of cranes and other marsh-birds, about the curvature of the cornea of the eye by which it is adapted to distinct perception in very different circumstances, and about the vocal organs of singing birds and of other animals in general.

But can we assume an unlimited extension of this " auto-plasmation " ? Is it possible to assume it in the case of the first formation of bones ? Our author maintains that when mineral salts are more abundantly deposited in the intercellular substance, the animal must experience the greater resistance to deformation which the tissue acquires thereby and that it can thus judge of the capacity of this means, constituted by the presence of these salts in its circulatory fluids, of satisfying the need experienced of a greater resistance in certain parts of the body. Now we hardly think that many people will be disposed to admit that even if the animal had had this experience as a result of a hypothetical magnified sensitivity, it could have succeeded by its effort in increasing the deposit of mineral matter in the necessary places.

Pauly, indeed, goes so far as to maintain that every need felt by the animal as a whole is transmitted to its smallest parts, and that consequently each of these parts is rendered capable of feeling the want of choosing the necessary means for its satisfaction, and that it can then perform the appropriate actions. But can such assumptions be really regarded as a serious attempt at explanation ?

Pauly's theory therefore must be classed with theories which we may term vitalistico-animistic even if they do not include any definitely religious elements. All these theories agree in assuming, as a fundamental characteristic of vital energy, not some simple and elementary properties similar to those of other forms of energy even if variable from one type of energy to another, but one extraordinary very complicated quality more or less similar to the reason of man.

We shall certainly not be deterred from considering Pauly as an animist by the fact that, after involving himself ever deeper in metaphysical obscurity, he finally attributes this property of intelligence to all energy and in this way imagines that he can resolve the old dualism between living and dead matter. But it is useless to stop to discuss this mere play of words. It is more useful to draw attention to the fact that at the present time we can observe everywhere a marked revival of these vitalistico-animistic ideas and the favourable reception which has been accorded to Pauly's work is a conspicuous testimony to the reality of this revival.

This revival, we must admit has been the result of the utter impotence of purely mechanical or physico-chemical theories to give any reasonable explanation of numerous essential features of vital phenomena, especially of those which in marked degree give evidence of purpose. They cannot explain onto-genetic development in which organs are formed which are adapted to the performance of functions which they will only accomplish in the adult, nor can they account for the activities of animals and plants which undeniably strive to accomplish ends which can only be achieved in a more or less distant future.

If our only difficulty was to account for the property which organisms possess of adapting themselves at every moment to continually changing external circumstances, we could select a large number of instances from the inorganic world which appear to be, in certain respects, of similar though not identical nature. For indeed every physico-chemical system, if its dynamic equilibrium be disturbed by external forces, tends to settle down into a new condition of dynamic equilibrium—that is " to adapt itself " to new external circumstances.

No one, we imagine, would become excited in contemplating the power of " adapting itself to an end " (" Zweckmässigkeit ") possessed by the flowing water in a river, which accumulates behind the piers of a bridge to such an extent as to produce the pressure necessary to increase the rapidity of flow so that the same quantity of water passes in a given time as passed in the same time before the bridge was built. For in this case it is obvious that what brings about the passage from a condition of disturbance to a new condition of equilibrium is just the fact that the current cannot stop, but is forced to continue to flow in the same volume. It is indeed the very obstacle which opposes the natural flow of the current which brings about the conditions (raising the water-level above the bridge) required to establish a new dynamic equilibrium and to accelerate the rapidity of flow which it should apparently retard.

We might make the same assertion about the electrical energy which passes between two metallic plates embedded in the earth and maintained at a constant difference of potential from one another. When the dynamic equilibrium of this flow is disturbed by a greater dryness of the air which causes too rapid evaporation and makes the superficial layer of the soil into a bad conductor, the electric energy is forced to pass through deeper layers of the ground. So, too, we may take the case of the chemical energy released by the strong affinity of two elements for each other. When the two compounds, each containing one of these elements, are dissolved, the multiple reactions which result from the mixture of these solutions are modified by a lowering of temperature which slows down or even reverses some of the secondary reactions. In these cases also we find that the electrical energy or chemical energy continues to be produced, and that it is just for this reason that the obstacle to its passage or to its production, creates the very conditions necessary for the establishment of a new equilibrium.

In the same way, if we assume that within certain limits of variation of the environment vital energy is unable to stop, but goes on being continually produced, and, moreover, that the tendency of living substance to increase continually in amount is the result of a corresponding irresistible tendency to expansion in vital energy, resulting from definite transformations of energy, then every obstacle which within these limits opposes the vital process will produce the new conditions (if necessary by stimulating the vital process itself) capable of establishing a new dynamic equilibrium, which is really an adaptation to the new environment.

Thus, though we are still unable completely to explain them, certain facts will no longer appear to us as the results of mysterious properties of living substance, as for instance, the fact that when tissues are submitted to pressure or traction, these influences, which perhaps at first constitute hindrances to the continuance of the vital process, may become changed into genuine " trophic stimuli " (Roux), as we learn from the structure of bones and the enlargement of the stalks of heavy fruits, or from the other fact that when the superficial layers of the skins of animals or of leaves are subjected to too great evaporation by being transported to a drier climate, or when they are transferred to colder conditions, they can resist and become adapted even to these unfavourable conditions of the environment by corresponding modifications of their vital processes.

But what these mechanical and physico-chemical analogies are unable to explain even in outline is the power of anticipation by which an organism prepares to accommodate itself to conditions not yet realised.

We must, therefore, assume the existence of a new property quite peculiar to vital energy. This property would consist in the circumstance that every state of physiological equilibrium as it gives place to a new one always leaves a trace of itself behind. This trace would consist of an accumulation of a corresponding specific variety of vital energy in each of the points of the organism which have been the seat of this physiological process now replaced by a new one. It follows that the return to activity of the physiological system No. 1 might be produced by the recurrence of a portion, perhaps even a small one, of the environmental conditions in response to which this physiological system was originally constituted.

This power of " releasing " an ancient physiological system by the reproduction of only a portion of the environmental conditions which originally determined its first appearance, is just this primordial fundamental " mnemonic " property of living substance which, as we have already seen, it is pre-eminently the

138

merit of Hering and Semon to have forced on our attention. It is this property which gives to all vital phenomena, from those of memory in the narrower sense down to and including all physiological phenomena, especially those of development, the appearance of preparations for environmental conditions which are not as yet completely realised. It is just this preparation for future conditions which constitutes the purposeful character of all vital phenomena and of psychic acts.

We see, therefore, that besides the alternative of purely mechanical physico-chemical theories, and of vitalistico-animistic conceptions, there is room for a third hypothesis which we have endeavoured to set forth in detail in the preceding chapters and which, for want of a better name, we may call the vitalistico-energetic theory. According to this theory, vital energy, which is perhaps merely nervous energy, though it is subject to the general laws of energetics, is characterised by quite peculiar qualities, so that it differs from other forms of energy, just as these differ from each other ; these qualities are, however, of a simple elementary nature, capable of being clearly defined, just like those of so-called physico-chemical forms of energy.

This theory, although it does not afford an explanation in the strict sense of the word of the phenomena of life, such as would allow of more extended and precise prediction of their course, may nevertheless suggest a new point of view, which might direct research in a different and more promising direction from that suggested by mechanical and physico-chemical views, which biologists have so far followed. Perhaps such researches, by striving to define clearly the properties which vital energy shares with other forms of energy and those by which it is distinguished from them, may succeed one day in finally terminating the age-long controversy between vitalists and materialists.

CHAPTER VIII

THE MNEMONIC BASIS OF THE PURPOSEFULNESS (FINALISM) OF LIFE ([1])

One of the most characteristic features of the purposefulness of life is exhibited by the " affective " impulses (affectivities). The fundamental tendency of the organism to maintain unchanged its physiological condition. Hunger and thirst. The environmental optimum. The urge to elimination. Sexual desire. The instinct of self-preservation. Quinton's theory compared with ours. Organic tendencies acquired during the lifetime of the individual which are doubtless of a mnemonic nature. It follows that inborn organic tendencies have also a mnemonic character. " Diffuse " seat of the " affective " tendencies and their property of being subjective (i.e. different from individual to individual). Special affective impulses which are developed through acquired habits. Maternal love. Family affection. The indispensability of the habitual. " Nature " is nothing but a " first habit." The law of the transferability and composition of the affective impulses will explain, if we grant the existence of a primitive stock of elementary affectivities, the whole range and the gradations of the sentiments of man.

BEFORE approaching the subject of the purposefulness or finalism of life, the philosophic importance of which is very great, we may take a backward glance over the road we have already traversed. In the earlier chapters we were concerned chiefly, though not exclusively, with ontogenic purposefulness, which is only one aspect of the general problem. It was in order to explain this ontogenic purposefulness, by

Thi s chapter was originally delivered as an address entitled "The purposefulness of life," to the College of France, on April 24th, 1920.

means of the transmissibility of acquired characters, that we elaborated our centro-epigenetic hypothesis, which, as we have seen, is fundamentally a mnemonic theory. We have now to consider the purposefulness of life in all its aspects. And, first of all, we shall show that this mnemonic property, to which we had recourse in our centro-epigenetic hypothesis, explains at the same time another manifestation—one of the most characteristic—of the purposefulness of life ; that is to say, it also explains the origin and nature of the " effective tendencies," as I shall term them. This will form the subject matter of the present chapter ; and in the chapter which follows it (IX) I shall take the opportunity offered by certain fundamental considerations, which may be deduced from certain characteristic properties of the affective tendencies, to examine the question of the purposefulness of life in the most general possible way.

If we examine the mode of action or the " behaviour " of various organisms from the protists to man, we see that a whole series of their actions, including the most essential, may be interpreted as instances of a tendency of the organism to maintain or to return to its " stationary " physiological state— using Ostwald's terminology in his writings on energetics. In other words, if we use the term " affective " to denote that special category of organic impulses which subjectively appear in our experience as " desires," " appetites " and " wants," and which objectively are manifested as non-mechanical movements, either actual or inceptive (i.e., in the nascent state), then we may consider all the principal "affective tendencies" as examples of the fundamental tendency of the organism to maintain its physiological condition unchanged.

We see, for instance, that the most fundamental "affective tendency" of all, viz., hunger, is in the final analysis nothing but an impulse to maintain or to restore in the internal nutritive medium the qualitative and quantitive conditions necessary for metabolism to persist in its "stationary" state. This is shown by the fact that once the condition of the internal nutritive medium has become normal, all desire on the part of the animal to seek additional nourishment *ipso facto* disappears.

Thus, a fresh-water polyp and a sea-anemone only react positively towards food if " their metabolism is in such a state as to require more material " (Jennings) ; so food placed on the disc of the large sea-anemone, *Stoichactis helianthus*, when the animal is not hungry, evokes the same characteristic "repulsive reaction" as does any deleterious substance. All organisms, from the top to the bottom of the scale of complexity of organisation, act in the same way.

The experiments of Schiff, who injected nutritive substances into the veins of a dog, prove in the clearest way that the essential nature of hunger is the impoverishment of the supply of histogenetic substances in the blood. For these injections not only nourished the dog but they also assuaged its hunger.

It follows obviously, we need scarcely say, that it is a matter of quite secondary importance that the feeling of hunger, when it is moderate, takes the form of a sensation localised in the wall of the stomach, which impels the animal to the same actions as those dictated by true hunger. This is only a case of the vicarious action of a part as representative of the whole, which characterises all mnemonic processes ; and this is true for the tendency to physiological stability, which is also, as we shall see later, of a mnemonic nature. These sensations, localised in the mucous membrane of the stomach, and due to the distension of its cells, or to some other similar change caused by the empty condition of the cavity, owing to the circumstance that they ordinarily precede and accompany the serious diminution of the histogenetic substances of the blood, eventually become the vicarious and representative manifestations of the deficiency of these substances.

The same explanation can be given of thirst and its apparent localisation in the upper parts of the digestive tube.

We might now pass from the consideration of hunger and thirst to that of other fundamental " appetites " or " needs." All these, by their manifestations, would reveal to us that their sole purpose is to re-establish the normal physiological condition, which in some way has been destroyed or disturbed.

So for each kind of animal there is an optimum environment as regards the concentration of the solution in which the animal lives, or the temperature of the medium, or the intensity of illumination, above, or below the level of which the organism can no longer maintain its normal physiological condition, and which it strives at all costs to maintain. We see, for instance, that at a temperature of 28° C., Paramecium reacts negatively to a rise of temperature, whilst at 22° C., it reacts negatively to a fall of temperature. So also Euglena, in moderate illumination, reacts negatively to a diminution of luminosity, whereas when it is exposed to light of great intensity, it acts in the exactly contrary manner.

In these cases and others the tendency to maintain the normal physiological condition is changed into a tendency to maintain the stability of the medium enveloping the organism, whether this be an external or internal medium. Thus oysters and sea-anemones exposed to the air shut up, in a word, they behave in such a way as to preserve their typical internal condition of humidity unchanged. Under the category of stability of environment must be included also the position of the organism in relation to the various forces acting on it, and above all the force of gravity. From the tendency to maintain this relationship unchanged is derived the effort of the organism to preserve or to re-establish its proper position in space. Thus Amœba usually retracts its pseudopodia when these come into contact with solid non-edible substances ; but when it is suspended in mid-water, it extends its pseudopodia in all directions, and as soon as it has succeeded in touching a solid body with one of them, it attaches itself to this and draws its whole body in this direction, and so restores its old relation to the substratum.

A star-fish, when placed upside down, strives to "right" itself—that is to return to its normal environmental conditions with respect to gravity.

Again, the need of eliminating the substances produced by metabolism, which the organism can no longer make use of, can be comprised in the same category, whether we are dealing with the lowest infusorian or with the most complicated vertebrate. For the feeling of the " need " of getting rid of these substances, although it may be evoked by local sensations which act as stimulants to the performance of the eliminatory act, is in the last resort due to the fact that the accummulation of the products of destructive metabolism in the interior of the animal would disturb its normal physiological state.

To this subdivision of eliminatory " affective " tendencies seems to belong also the sexual " instinct " or " hunger." There is a tendency nowadays to regard this " sexual hunger," like ordinary hunger, as having its seat not in the localised region, such as the genital organs, but in the entire organism, and to suggest as the ultimate cause of the sexual instinct the need experienced of getting rid of the germinal substance. According to this view, " sexual hunger " would be nothing but the effort of the organism to get rid of the physiological disturbance produced by the germinal substance, this disturbance being a result of the abnormal and unstable condition of the nuclear substance of the germinal cells, reduced to a half, and ripe for fertilisation, and of its slow disintegration, which acts as an irritating hormonic secretion, diffusing itself throughout the entire organism.

The more or less brilliant " nuptial livery," with which nearly all animals are clothed at the time of mating, is there to denote what an abnormal condition of hypersecretion is caused by these hormonic dis-integrative products of the germinal substance, and to indicate what a profound physiological disturbance of all the cells of the body is caused by it.

The impulse to eliminate such a profoundly dis-turbing substance would subsequently become an impulse towards sexual union as the proper means of effecting this elimination.

It follows that, as Ribot justly remarks, sexual love is fundamentally egoistic. He says: " In the vast majority of animals the sexual instinct is not accompanied by any tender emotion. Once the sexual act is accomplished, separation and obliviscence supervene."

This theory which gives to the sexual instinct merely the significance of the impulse to eliminate an irritating substance, allows us to view this instinct in a very different light from that in which it has until now been considered. If the theory is accepted it would not be for the " good " of the species, but solely for that of the individual that the sexual instinct had been evolved and had developed. It could no longer be regarded as the " will of the species " im-posing itself on the individual, as many with Schopen-hauer still continue to believe, but rather in this case, as in all others, the " will " of the individual itself — that is the normal impulse of the individual to maintain its normal physiological condition unchanged.

Once we have succeeded in referring the sexual instinct to the category of impulses seeking to maintain unchanged the normal stationary physiological state of the organism, this law is found to hold good, without exception, for all the " affective tendencies." We can therefore briefly formulate it in the following words. Each organism is a physiological system in a stationary (stable) condition and strives to maintain that condition, or to restore it every time that it is disturbed by a change supervening in either the external or internal environment. This property is the basis of all the most essential organic " needs " and " appetites." All movements of approach or retreat, of attack or flight, of capture or rejection, carried out by animals are only so many direct or indirect consequences of this general tendency of each " stationary " physiological state to maintain itself unchanged. We shall see later how this tendency is related to the fundamental mnemonic property of all living substance.

This sole generalised physiological tendency will account for a whole series of the most varied special " affective tendencies." Thus every special cause of disturbance will produce a corresponding impulse of repulsion with its own peculiar characteristics determined by the nature of the disturbance, by its intensity and by the means which it is necessary to adopt in order to evade the disturbance, and for each factor capable of preserving the normal physiological condition or restoring it, we shall have a corresponding and distinct impulse of " longing," " desire," " attraction " and so forth.

The " instinct of self-preservation," in the narrower sense of the preservation of the life of the individual, is also only a special derivative and direct consequence of this general tendency to the preservation of the normal physiological state, since it is obvious that every situation which finally becomes fatal is at first a mere disturbance, and it is under this aspect that the animal strives and learns to escape from it. Thus the Amœba of Jennings which was completely swallowed by another Amœba and strove to escape and ultimately succeeded in doing so, did not act to avoid a factor which endangered its life, but merely to escape from a situation which was profoundly disturbing.

Quinton, as is well-known, was the first to develop a theory of the tendency of organisms to maintain their own internal environment in the same physico-chemical conditions which prevailed when life first appeared on the earth. But the theory which we have just set forth limits itself, as we have seen, to dealing with this tendency to stability which is manifested every moment in the mode of " behaviour " of each individual. Instead of serving as a doubtful point of departure, as does the theory of Quinton, for a theory of the evolution of species, it forms a solid basis from which it is possible to derive all the " affective tendencies " of the animal world.

Though it is a factor of stability as regards the individual, this tendency towards physiological invariability has become one of the principal factors in variation and progress, so far as the species is concerned, but in quite another sense than that indicated by Quinton ; it is because it has aroused and developed the power of movement, which constitutes the greatest distinction, though it is not an absolute one, between the animal and vegetable worlds, and because the development of this power has entailed the development and improvement of all the locomotor apparatus and of the nervous system correlated therewith, the different forms of which constitute a large proportion of the fundamental characteristics which distinguish the various kinds of animals from one another.

Finally, this universal tendency to stability so far as the individual is concerned, has become in man one of the principal factors in all social evolution. For we can see that all technical inventions, and the whole of economic production have had and still have, directly or indirectly, one single purpose, from the first dwellings of the troglodytes, the use of skins as clothing and the discovery of fire, up to the greatest refinements of our time, and that aim has been, and is, to maintain by artificial means the greatest possible stability of the environment as a necessary and sufficient condition for preserving the physiological invariability.

In addition to the fundamental property possessed by all organisms of striving each to maintain its normal physiological condition unchanged and to restore it when it is disturbed, they possess another property which in its turn has given rise to new " affectivities."

For when the former " stationary " physiological state can be no longer restored by the use of any device—that is to say, by any form of movement—the organism tends to pass into a new " stationary " state which is compatible with the new internal or external environment. Thus arise a new set of phenomena termed " phenomena of adaptation."

For instance the classical experiments of Dallinger on the acclimatisation of the lower organisms have proved that infusoria can be gradually accustomed to endure successively higher temperatures, and after a year of such graduated increases of temperature they succeed in living under conditions which would kill a similar organism which had not been acclimatised. Similarly we know that the same species of protozoa occur both in fresh and salt water, and that it is possible gradually to accustom the amœbæ and infusoria of fresh water to live in water of a degree of salinity which would at first have destroyed them ; and many other examples of similar new adaptations could be given.

Now what is interesting to note is that the new environmental conditions, to which the animal gradually becomes accustomed, finally become for it optimum condition. " Individual adaptation," writes Dallinger (as for instance, to a new condition of salinity), " takes place according to the law that the conditions of density under which an individual is forced to live, tend to become in time the most favourable conditions for that individual."

The truth of this law can be proved even for vegetable organisms.

Thus plasmodia of Myxomycetes, which would succumb if suddenly placed in solutions of glucose of a strength of 2 per cent. and which retire from solutions of $\frac{1}{2}$ or even $\frac{1}{4}$ per cent., can be gradually accustomed to live in solutions of 2 per cent. and show by their behaviour that they prefer these to weaker solutions. The diatom *Navicula brevis* normally avoids light of even minimum intensity, but diatoms in a culture which had been previously exposed for several weeks to the full light of a window, tended to accumulate in the best lighted portion of a drop of water when this drop was replaced in the primitive obscurity.

The common sea-anemone (*Actinia equina*) which is found attached to rocks in every conceivable position with regard to the vertical—with the axis of the body directed upwards, downwards or horizontally, seems to become so much accustomed to its particular position that when it is removed from its support it tends to revert to its old position. Thus when sea anemones, attached in all sorts of positions, are collected and put into an aquarium, " we can observe," writes M. Piéron, " a tendency amongst them in seeking new attachments to assume the same position (with regard to the vertical) as that which they previously occupied."

We could give numerous other examples of similar phenomena, but the important point is to emphasise their significance. They prove that the new physiological condition which constitutes the adaptation of the organism to the new environment, once it has been established and has lasted some time, tends to restore itself. Now this tendency to its own " reactivation " or reproduction which is thus manifested by every former physiological state is nothing else than the tendency to its own " evocation " shown by every mnemonic accumulation, and is therefore of a purely mnemonic character.

Consequently there follows a deduction of even greater importance, which is that we must attribute a similar mnemonic nature to this fundamental tendency to preserve physiological stability whence we have derived all the most fundamental " affective tendencies " of all organisms without exception. In fact, if in the cases which we have mentioned, a quite new and recently acquired physiological state is able to deposit a mnemonic accumulation of itself sufficiently strong to ensure its own revival, we can easily understand how the normal physiological state, by reason of its immensely longer duration, should manifest a much more powerful mnemonic tendency to re-establish itself when it is disturbed.

This implies that all the numberless elementary physiological states in various points of the body, which together make up the general physiological state of the whole, have each the power of depositing its own specific accumulation, just as everything leads us to suppose that the nervous currents passing in the brain, which give rise to the varied sensations, leave behind them similar mnemonic deposits which can cause the revival of these sensations. By the phrase " specific accumulation," we mean only this, that each accumulation, by its discharge, gives rise to exactly the same specific variety of nervous current, by the action of which as " charging current " it was deposited.

The extension of this power of specific accumulation to all physiological phenomena, is in harmony with the theory which regards nervous energy as the basis of all vital phenomena.

There would only be this difference, that in psychic memory in the narrower sense, the phenomena of the excitation or discharge of the nervous energy are prominently in the foreground, whilst the special physico-chemical phenomena, accompanying this nervous discharge, recede into the background, so that until quite recently they were completely ignored, and that amongst physiological phenomena exactly the reverse happens, but the difference is one of degree, and not of nature.

Claude Bernard maintains in fact that " all forms of irritability of living substance are essentially identical in their nature." If, then, along with the physico-chemical phenomena accompanying the activation, for instance, of both muscular tissue and glandular cells, the comcomitant specific nervous phenomena are less easily perceptible, this is no reason to doubt their existence.

As a consequence of this extension of the mnemonic property to all the elementary physiological processes we obtain a *somatic or visceral theory of the fundamental " affective tendencies."* By this we mean that the tendency both to maintain unchanged the normal physiological state, and to re-establish a given physiological state corresponding to a former environment, is due to a whole mass of elementary specific accumulations, which, varying in their specific nature from point to point of the body, constitute, taken together, a sum of potential energy acting like a force of gravitation towards the medium or environment, which either tends to maintain or to restablish the whole physiological state represented by these elementary accumulations.

THE PURPOSEFULNESS OF LIFE

Of course, in organisms provided with a nervous system, side by side with each of these " affective tendencies " of purely somatic origin and seat, there will gradually be added a co-operative and vicarious " tendency," due to mnemonic deposits in that particular part of the nervous system which is in direct relation with the part of the body where the visceral " affective tendency " originates. In man this part will be Flechsig's " area of visceral sensation " (*Körperfühlsphäre*) in the brain, to which in certain cases the frontal region of the cortex is added.

There are, therefore, two fundamental properties which the affective tendencies derive from their mnemonic visceral origin, viz. : (1) that of having a diffuse seat, that is of being diffuse in their localisation, and (2) that of being " subjective " (personal), that is of varying from individual to individual.

The first property is due to the fact that every physiological state affects every point in the body, or in that large part of the body in which it is established, and consequently affects also all the numberless points of that part of the brain in which the corresponding part of the organism is, so to speak, reflected. Whilst, therefore, we have every reason to believe that each sensory mnemonic accumulation has its seat in a sole point, or, at most, in a narrowly limited area of the cerebral cortex, we are equally justified, on the other hand, in supposing that each " affective tendency " is made up of an infinite number of elementary mnemonic accumulations deposited in each point of the body and in each corresponding point of the brain.

As regards the second property of the affective

BIOLOGICAL MEMORY

tendencies, viz., that of being subjective or personal, this is due to the fact that the organism will be endowed with certain idiosyncrasies, and with certain longings (nostalgia), according to the various environments or situations to which the individual or the species has been exposed in the past for a sufficient length of time, that is to say, according to *the particular history* in each case. So we can understand the subjectivity and the infinite variety which are manifested in all the wants, appetites, and desires, and in all that becomes the subject of affective judgment.

In support of the hypothesis of the mnemonic nature of all the affective tendencies which we have just set forth, we might adduce examples of specialised affective tendencies which have arisen through habit. It will be sufficient to take as single instance of these tendencies, maternal love.

Evidently this is an example of the habit of parasitic relationship or of symbiosis, which from having been continued for many generations, has gradually become changed, by the mnemonic property, into an affective tendency towards those relations. As Giard says, " Comparative ethology shows us in the clearest manner that the relations between the parental organism and its offspring are fundamentally similar to those which subsist between a host and its parasite, and that after a period of instability, during which the one or the other organism suffers for the advantage of its companion, the relations between them attain a condition of mutual equilibrium."

For instance, if we consider the question of lactation,

156

we find that this began by the young ones sucking up the secretions of the sudoriferous glands in the breast of the mother which covered them, and that this habit has caused these glands to develop into milk-glands and has at the same time developed in the mother a veritable craving to be sucked. To quote Giard again, "Amongst mammals it is to the phenomena of lactation and suckling that we must look for the origins of the relations of mutual symbiosis which unite the mother and the child. The physiological disturbances of pregnancy and parturition entail, amongst other very curious results, a hypersecretion of the mammary glands which are only a local hypertrophy of the sebaceous glands of the skin. The young one by licking up and sucking this secretion, from which it derives its first nourishment, assuages the need experienced by the female to be sucked, and in this way it becomes for its mother a means of comfort."

That the need of being sucked is the origin of maternal love we see quite plainly from the fact that if a mother is deprived of her offspring, she feels the need of replacing them by other nurselings. " The need of ridding herself of an irritating secre-tion," writes Giard, " is sometimes so powerful as to induce the female deprived of her young to steal the offspring of another female, and these thefts of children have also been observed in females which were suckling their own children ; as very often happens, the satisfaction derived from assuaging a need had led them to seek still greater measures of this satisfaction, and even to go to excess. "

In the cases observed by Lloyd Morgan, this need of

the mother to give suck takes on the aspect of a tender solicitude for the nourishment of the young. " I have seen," he says, " both bitches and cats get up and again lie down so as to bring the teats into closer proximity to the mouth of any young one which failed to find them. When a lamb is weakly and fails to find the teat, the mother not infrequently uses its shoulders, head and neck as a lever to place the lamb on its legs, and having accomplished this, straddles over the lamb and brings the teats against its lips, and these efforts are continued until the little animal sucks."

This typical instance shows us clearly how the need of getting rid of the milk has led to an affective attraction towards the young one as the customary means of eliminating this fluid, in the same way that the desire to eliminate the germinal substance, as we have seen above, has led to an affective attraction towards the opposite sex as affording the usual means of getting rid of this substance.

In point of fact, just as " sexual attraction " ceases, once the germinal substance has been got rid of, so " maternal affection," in the case of most mammals, ceases as soon as the need of getting rid of the milk comes to an end. " Maternal affection," observes Giard, " does not usually survive the causes which have brought it into being, and only obscure traces of it can be found once lactation has ceased."

Finally, the fact that maternal love is stronger than paternal love, and that the love of parents for their children is stronger than that of children for their parents, support the view that all these " affectivities " have originated as the result of habits ; for they demonstrate that these affectivities are proportionately stronger, according to the number and persistence of the relations from which they have originated. " In the animal kingdom in general," observes Ribot, " paternal love is rare and unstable, and amongst the lower representatives of humanity it is a very feeble emotion, and a very loose tie." It is only met with in the case of stable sexual unions, where the common life " has created a current of affection due to the mutual help which the partners render to each other."

" Everyone admits," says Pillon, " that the love of parents for their children exceeds in intensity the love of children for their parents, and if we compare the father and the mother, it is the latter that has most love for the child. The reason of this is that in the mother, as a result of her special functions, the love is nourished and increased—much more than it is in the case of the father—by the continuity of the acts to which love is due."

But maternal love and family love in general, originating as they do in certain relations which have become habitual, constitute only one particular instance of a very general law . Every other relation even if very specialised, which become established with things or persons, has no sooner become a habit than it becomes, in virtue of this very fact, a " need."

In a word, Lehmann's law of " the necessity of the habitual," which that author enunciated for every stimulus to which we become accustomed, and the cessation of which gives rise to a need, can be verified in the case of every relation to the environment, general or particular.

BIOLOGICAL MEMORY

" I have in my room," wrote a friend to G. E. Müller, " a clock which does not go for more than 24 hours without being rewound, and so it very often stops. When that occurs, I notice it at once, whereas, of course, I perceive nothing as long as the clock is going. When it stopped for the first time, this was the change which took place in me : I experienced all at once an indefinable uneasiness, a kind of emptiness without being able to discover the cause of it. It was only after some reflection that I found the cause in the stoppage of the clock."

Moreover, it is a familiar fact known to everybody, that habit can induce us to take pleasure in things which are at first disagreeable, and that certain habits which a man contracts during his life-time, become for him needs as imperious as the so-called natural ones. " Smokers, snuff-takers, and those who chew tobacco," writes Herbert Spencer, " furnish familiar instances of the way in which the long persistence in a sensation, not originally agreeable, makes it pleasurable, the sensation itself remaining unchanged. The like happens with various foods and drinks, which, at first distasteful, are afterwards greatly relished if frequently taken."

In this way the nostalgia (longing) for every customary thing which happens to be wanting, is originated. " There is produced," writes Ribot, " in certain animals a condition comparable to our nostalgia which manifests itself in a violent desire to return to places which they formerly inhabited, or by the pining away which results from the absence of people and of things to which they are accustomed."

Thus, for instance, persistent habit suffices to explain the origin and deeply engrained character in both animals and men of many affective tendencies, analogous to family affection, but of a far wider range such as gregariousness, sociability, friendship and so on. Spencer speaks thus of them: " The perception of kindred beings, perpetually seen, heard and smelt, will come to form a predominant part of consciousness, so predominant a part that the absence of it will inevitably cause discomfort."

From these few examples, which we have adduced as illustrations of our hypothesis, we see how profoundly true is the popular saying that " habit is second nature."

If, however, we have the opportunity of watching the most various kinds of " affectivities " originate before our eyes—so to speak—as the results of habit, we are justified in referring to mnemonic causes of the same kind, *all* the affective tendencies, without exception, for the nature of those that are inborn is exactly the same as the nature of those that are acquired ; just as Lamarckian evolutionists, arguing from cases of functional adaptation acquired during life which they have observed, legitimately deduce the conclusion that the whole general structure of the organism has been built up by a long series of similar functional adaptations.

We may thus supplement the popular saying that " habit is second nature," by adding, inversely, " nature is nothing but primordial habit."

There is another special property of " affective

tendencies," which, being essentially mnemonic in character, confirms their mnemonic origin and nature; it is what Ribot terms their power of "transference." In virtue of this property the affectivities of direct mnemonic origin give rise to secondary affectivities, which may thus be said to have an indirect mnemonic origin.

This property of "transference" consists in the vicarious substitution of the whole by a part. In virtue of this property, portions of a situation which in its totality has been previously an object of desire, or situations regarded as analogous to the desired one, or environmental relations which constitute suitable means for the accomplishment of the desired end, or, finally, environmental relations which have always been associated with this end, are able to awaken the same "affectivity" as the end itself.

This secondary affectivity at first awakened by the presence of a part as representative of the whole, comes in course of time, through habit, to be firmly attached to this part, which thenceforward becomes desired for itself, quite apart from its nature as a representative of the situation first desired only as a whole.

This is what occurs, as we have already indicated, with regard to the union of the two sexes—desired at first as a means of getting rid of germinal substances—and also with regard to the secondary sexual relations as customary phenomena associated with this union, both of which are now longed for, quite apart from the need of eliminating the disturbing germinal substance. The "conquest" of the opposite sex, which is indispensable for the satisfaction of "sexual hunger," eventually becomes in certain people an end in itself ; the delight in seduction for the sake of seduction, the sexual vanity of the male as well as of the female, and other similar affectivities are further derivatives of the sexual appetite.

The same thing is true of the action of a carnivorous animal in tearing its prey to pieces. This action begins by being the customary means of satisfying hunger, but it finally becomes a delight in cruelty for the sake of cruelty. " One half of the animal race," writes Bain, "lives upon prey ; and as it is delightful to eat, so it must be delightful to kill. Pleasurable must also be all the signs of discomfiture, the helpless struggles and agonised gestures of the victim."

As a result of further " transference," in the case of man, this struggle for life gave rise to the desire of victory for its own sake, the lust of domination, the greed of power, the passion of glory and of renown, and the ambition to excel above one's equals.

In this and many other similar cases of " transferred " affectivities from relations of a more material kind to those of less and less material and more and more moral nature, along with the " transference " in the narrower sense, which makes the part into a new object of desire, there has co-operated incessantly, in the higher animals and in man, their intellectual development.

Intelligence, in fact, by the power which it confers of a continually increasing capacity of predicting external phenomena, succeeds in discovering new methods, more and more complex and indirect of attaining certain ends, and thus it opens to the affective " transference " an ever widening field of action.

Arms, originally invented by man as a means of self-preservation, have attracted an " affective tendency " to themselves, typical of the warrior and of the hunter ; similarly the soil, the culture of which has become the principal means of obtaining food, has engendered that intense love of it, for its own sake, which is found among peasants.

Further, intelligence, by the ever increasing power which it confers of foreseeing internal psychic events, gives rise to a whole series of new affectivities, which express themselves as desires to prevent the eventual disappointment of future affectivities. Thus, for instance, the fear of future hunger gives rise, even in a satiated man, to an " affectivity " directed towards the preservation and retention in his own possession of stored food, and, as a consequence, to the general " sentiment of property," and to a thousand of other desires which civilised man experiences, and which develop in him in such an intense degree : the envy of riches, the greediness of lucre, and other similar sentiments.

Finally, it is intelligence which makes possible the infinite gradation of " shades " which may be manifested by the human affective tendencies. In virtue of the power which intelligence possesses of considering each environmental relation, as soon as it becomes slightly complicated, from several points of view nearly contemporaneously, it succeeds in awakening simultaneously numerous affectivities, and these, then,

THE PURPOSEFULNESS OF LIFE

by mutual union, composition, interference and inhibition, as Bain says, finally give rise to an exceedingly complex resultant affectivity, which according to the number and nature of its com‑ponents, can from one case to another, manifest the finest degrees of difference.

The instinct of self-preservation, for instance, had already developed in animals the sentiments of fear, of timidity, and similar affectivities. In man it gives rise to propitiatory affectivities of all degrees, such as those of self-prostration, humility, hypocrisy, adula-tion and so on. Religious feeling itself, in its lower forms, is directly derived from the propitiatory affectivity. The higher forms of religious feeling, such as are experienced in the contemplation of the sublime, are more highly developed forms of this affectivity.

From the same instinct of self-preservation, under its defensive and offensive forms, there had been already developed in all the higher animals, the impulse to attack and counter-attack. In man this impulse has assumed the most varied forms and varying degrees of development, from the feeling of deep hatred to that of scarcely perceptible dislike, from the lust of plunder to simple envy, from the most ferocious desire for revenge to the slightest resentment.

The lofty sentiment of " justice " itself is the distant and scarcely recognisable derivative of this sentiment of self-preservation.

Good examples of the high degree of complexity which can be obtained in this way are provided by maternal love, which beginning as the physical need of being sucked, develops into the most tender sentiments of a pure altruism, and especially by conjugal affection, which beginning in purely animal sexual hunger, rises to a harmonious sympathy of the sweetest and most delicate moral affectivities.

It will, however, be easily perceived that it is both useless and impossible to pursue further the analysis of all the affectivities, and of all their nuances which have ultimately originated and developed in the higher animals and, above all, in man.

We wish merely to point out, by this very summary review, that once the organism has acquired a stock of affective tendencies in a direct mnemonic fashion, and once the intelligence has been adequately developed, the number of further affective tendencies which can be derived from them by " transference " and " composition " is really infinite.

It is, of course, also needless to say to scientific men, and even to young students who have already imbibed the scientific spirit, that the lowly mnemonic origin of our most tender affectivities and of our highest aspirations, should in no way either shock us or stifle or diminish the intense internal impulse and spiritual struggle to attain higher and higher moral levels, which we all experience. On the contrary the recognition of the enormous extent to which our souls, starting from such humble origins, have been able to raise and purify themselves, should give to us the assurance of the possibility that they can be still further elevated and purified, and thus incite us to redouble our efforts to attain a still greater degree of

moral perfection, and a still further ascent towards the
ideal.

It remains for us, now that the mnemonic origin and
nature of all our affective tendencies has been demonstrated, to consider the consequences with regard to
the purposefulness, or finalism, of life in general,
which can be deduced therefrom. And this we shall
do in the following chapter.

CHAPTER IX

THE MNEMONIC BASIS OF THE PURPOSEFULNES OF LIFE (*Continued*)

The fundamental property of " affective tendencies " is to strive to reach an end without at first any preference for the route to be followed. The fundamental difference between the mechanical reflex on the one hand, which is discharged along a single determinate path, and the affective tendency on the other, which constitutes a force in which neither the point of application nor the path are determined, but only the end to be reached. The end which a given affective tendency strives to reach, manifests itself as a " pull from in front " (*vis a fronte*), or final cause, of an entirely different nature from the " push from behind " (*vis a tergo*), or actual cause, which alone is met with in the inorganic world. It is the mnemonic accumulations, which the physiological activities which have been produced in the past by the action of the medium towards which the animal is now striving, have left behind them, which constitute the true and effective "*vis a tergo*" which moves the living organism. Consequently, this mnemonic property appears to be completely adequate to explain also all the purposefulness (finalism) of life. It is because it is wanting in the inorganic realm that this realm is devoid of all appearance of purposefulness. This contrast between our inner life which is steeped in purposefulness and the inanimate external universe in which we can detect no trace of purpose, constitutes the underlying basis of the age-long strife between science and religion.

IF in the preceding chapter we have succeeded in demonstrating the direct or indirect mnemonic origin and nature of all the affective tendencies, we can deduce from this thesis most important consequences as regards the purposefulness of life.

Let us first consider the fundamental character of the affective tendencies, viz., that they are forces striving to reach definite ends, but leaving indeterminate the route to be followed.

THE PURPOSEFULNESS OF LIFE—(cont.)

This property of striving towards an end, without any preference for the particular means chosen to reach it, so characteristic of the affective tendencies, is due to the existence in a potential condition of the definite physiological condition, general or partial, the re-awakening of which constitutes the sole and real end. This mnemonic accumulation is, as we have seen in the preceding chapter, the trace left behind by a re-action of the organism, either to the whole environment or to some particular elements of it, and it tends now, like every other kind of potential energy, once it is " released " by the persistence or return of the old environment, or of some part of it, to become again kinetic. In a word, the existence of the affective tendency results only in impelling the organism towards the medium or the environmental relations which permit the corresponding physiological condition again to become active ; but this " impulsion " does not in itself involve a preference for one set of movements rather than another, any one of which might eventually prove able to bring back the organism to the medium it strives for, *but none of which, nevertheless, have anything in common with the definitive physiological condition which tends again to become active.* It is only when a series of movements has succeeded by chance better than others in restoring the organism to the desired environmental conditions, that from that time on it will be preferred to the others ; which is expressed by the statement that the affectivity has made *a choice* (William James, Baldwin and all the American School).

This amounts to saying that it is only from this time

on, that the affectivity will become by mnemonic association an " impulsion " towards a given series of movements which bring about the desired end, in the same way as certain reflexes impinge upon one another (Sherrington). Consequently it will only be from this time that these movements will be constantly repeated, under the influence of the affective tendency, until they are " mechanised " in the form of reflexes.

But until this point is reached, the affective tendency is not impelled to discharge itself in one way rather than in another. So it follows that the great difference between the affective tendency on the one hand and the reflex on the other hand is just this, that the latter—in which the " chosen " act, often repeated, tends to become " mechanised " and autonomous—represents a tendency towards a discharge along a predetermined path. It becomes a force of which the point of application and the direction are known beforehand, and which can consequently be graphically represented by the customary arrow which is used to denote ordinary mechanical forces. The affective tendency on the other hand is a force of which neither the point of application nor the direction are determined beforehand, but solely the point which it strives to reach. It is a fund of available energy which can be applied indifferently to one action or to another, provided that the action is adapted to attain the desired end. It can therefore be represented by any one of an infinite number of arrows filling a conical space and all converging towards the apex of the cone.

A reflex tendency, consequently, only admits of a

single solution ; an affective tendency on the other hand, so long as none of the possible movements performed by chance has succeeded and has given rise to a choice, or so long as many equivalent routes of reaching the end are available, is capable of a large and indefinite number of solutions.

It is this possibility of numerous alternative solutions which constitutes the unforeseen, the anti-mechanistic character of affective behaviour, as compared with the pre-determined and mechanical behaviour of the reflex or of every combination of reflexes, however complicated, like certain instincts.

Finally, it is this fundamental character of an affective tendency, namely, that it acts like a force of gravitation directed towards the medium or the particular environmental relations which allow of the entry into activity of the mnemonic deposits constituting the particular tendency, which gives to the medium, or the environmental relations, the appearance of pull from in front (*vis a fronte*) or "final cause," of totalling different nature from the ordinary *vis a tergo*, or " actual cause," which alone is operative in the inorganic world. " The organism," writes Jennings, " seems to work towards a definite end. In other words, the final result of its action seems to be present in some way at the beginning, deter-mining what the action shall be. In this the action of living things appears to contrast with that of things inorganic."

Now we see that this final result of the action is really present from the beginning in the form of a mnemonic accumulation : the medium, or the environmental relations towards which the animal strives, operate now like a *vis a fronte* solely because they have formerly been a *vis a tergo*, and because the physiological activities which they have then aroused in the organism have left behind them a mnemonic deposit, which now acts like a veritable *vis a tergo* in moving the living being.

Thus the same explanation is seen to be valid for all the finalism of life.

Every manifestation of purposefulness, from onto-genetic development, which builds up organs which can only be used in the adult state, to the property of physiological states in general, corresponding to certain environmental conditions, to become active at the first appearance of phenomena which ordinarily precede, but do not constitute, the whole of these environmental conditions ; from the perfect morpho-logical adaptation of the organism to the environment, completed before the environment has been able to exert its formative action, to the wonderful arrange-ments and specialised structures so nicely calculated in view of certain probable conditions to which, in the future, the organism may be exposed ; from simple reflex actions " mechanised " for the purpose of the preservation and prosperity of the individual to all the most complex instincts by which animals provide beforehand for future conditions of which they know nothing : all these purposeful aspects of life can be explained, as has been set forth in our works cited above and partially in the preceding chapters of this book, as so many manifestations of mnemonic nature.

Now we have seen that the affective tendencies themselves, which are the most prominently purposeful of all vital phenomena, can also be derived from the mnemonic property of living substance, that is in the last resort from the power of specific accumulation, which is found only in nervous energy, the basis of all life.

" Mnemonic property," " power of specific accumulation," these by their absence from the inorganic world leave it completely to the mercy of the " *a tergo* " forces, and deprive it of all appearance of purpose ; by their presence in the organic realm they make it a world in itself, whose peculiarities the physico-chemical laws interpreted in the narrow sense customary to-day, are totally inadequate to explain.

So there is generated the tragic and eternal opposition between our inner life which is steeped in purpose, and which feels purpose to be the very marrow of its bones, and the external inorganic world which, though it has been anxiously scrutinised for numberless centuries, seems to us to show no trace of purpose at all. It is this tragic and eternal opposition between the purposeful microcosm and the purely mechanical macrocosm which constitutes the ground of the age-long strife between science and religion, the first, forced by reasoning based on facts to deny the existence of purpose in the universe, the second, irresistibly driven to affirm the presence of purpose by the deepest feelings of ourselves.

This struggle between reason and feeling will perhaps never come to an end, unless man determines to seek, only within the restricted circle of the world of life with which he has kinship of birth and nature, for the final reason of his conduct and the supreme purpose of his existence. And this kinship of origin and nature, if it is thoroughly grasped, will not fail to imbue man with a feeling of sympathy towards every kind of being which can enjoy and suffer, and in particular with a feeling of love and devotion towards the human family, which constitutes the apex of organic evolution, and in which the pulse of life throbs most actively and consciously. So man will be induced to combat everywhere by deeds of goodness and justice every cause of pain, and to assist every cause of gladness, since the first is a diminution and the second an enhancement of vital activity. He will be led to encourage, at the same time, all forms of social progress, all manifestations of beauty, all efforts towards the ideal, so that human life may roll on, becoming more and more complete, more and more serene, and more and more elevated, and that the torch of life may scatter into the universe ever more beams of brighter and purer light.

CHAPTER X

The criticism of our mnemonic theory of the purposefulness (finalism) of life put forward by Prof. Bottazzi, one of the most authoritative representatives of physico-chemical materialism. Prof. Bottazzi asserts that he has no knowledge of "nervous energy" and that the statement that this energy is the basis of life conveys no meaning to him. He admits that physiologists are ignorant of the physiological basis of the mnemonic faculty, but he maintains that non-living colloidal systems also manifest clear mnemonic properties. He raises the objection that what organisms strive to preserve is not a determinate physiological state, but just simply equilibrium as do all inorganic systems. His comparison of the organism with a vessel in which is contained a mixture of non-living materials developing a gas, and which has a valve permitting this gas to escape when it exceeds a certain pressure. According to the opinion of Prof. Bottazzi, we ought to cease to attribute purposefulness to the phenomena of life; purposefulness is a peculiar attitude of our own mind and does not correspond to the reality of the facts.

HAVING reached this point in our exposition of the mnemonic theory of life, it seems appropriate to examine the objections to this theory which have been raised by the partisans of physico-chemical theories of life and to learn what explanation these gentlemen have to offer of the purposefulness or finalism of life, the explanation of which we, for our part, consider is only to be found in the mnemonic properties of living substance. With this object we

175

shall select the criticism of our mnemonic theory of the purposefulness of life put forward by Prof. Filippo Bottazzi, of the University of Naples, who is one of the most authoritative and inflexible representatives of physico-chemical materialism. We shall give his criticism in its entirety and in his own words :

"Every living organism considered as a stationary system shows, according to the hypothesis advanced by Prof. Rignano in his essay on the purposefulness of life, a general tendency to preserve its physiological stability, that is its normal state ; consequently it tends to return to this state after each disturbance which occurs in the environment, exterior or interior. This property constitutes the basis of all the fundamental organic 'needs' and 'appetites.' It gives rise to and explains the most varied series of special affective tendencies—such as 'hunger,' 'thirst,' 'sexual desire,' etc., and the actions which aim at satisfying these needs.

"Moreover, when the original stationary normal state can no longer be restored in any way because of the impossibility of returning to the old environment, the organism tends to acquire a new stationary physiological state compatible with the new environment, that is to say, the organism manifests the so-called phenomena of adaptation ; and when adaptation has been attained, that is to say, when the organism has passed into the new stationary physiological state and has maintained itself in this state for some time, it tends to remain in it as if this state were indeed 'second nature' for it.

"Now this tendency, whether the physiological state

is an original or a secondarily acquired condition, can in turn be explained by an alleged fundamental mnemonic property of all living substance. This tendency to the revival or reproduction of a former physiological state—Rignano asserts—is only the tendency to become active which is possessed by every mnemonic accumulation. The mnemonic property is thus extended to all the elementary physiological processes, and in this way we obtain a somatic or visceral theory of the fundamental affective tendencies.

"These tendencies have a common fundamental character, which is to act like a force striving to attain an end, but leaving the path to that end indeterminate. This fundamental character of the affective tendency to act like a force of gravitation towards the medium or certain relations with the medium which will allow the mnemonic accumulations which make up the tendency, again to become active, is what gives to the environment, or to certain aspects of it, the appearance of a *'vis a fronte'* or 'final cause,' of quite a different nature from the ordinary *'vis a tergo'* or actual cause, which alone operates in the inorganic world.

"It is these affective tendencies, together with other fundamental phenomena of the organic world examined in detail by Rignano in his previous works, which give to the phenomena of life their appearance of purposefulness. Since all these phenomena are due to the fundamental mnemonic property of living substance—that is to say, in the last resort, to the power of specific accumulation, which is the peculiarity of that nervous energy which forms the basis of all the phenomena of the organic world—thus this mnemonic property of nervous energy will suffice to explain all the purposefulness of life.

"Such is, in brief summary, the very interesting address delivered by Prof. Rignano to the Athenaeum of Geneva on the 20th of April, and to the College of France on the 24th April, 1920.

"We cannot assume that a scientific man of the worth and attainments of Prof. Rignano could imagine that all the readers of his address would agree with what he has said on the phenomena of life. This disagreement of many with him will arise not only from general considerations, since vital phenomena are not regarded in the same manner by the physiologist and by the philosopher of nature, but also from special considerations.

"If we briefly refer to some of the latter, I should say for my own part that I am not acquainted with 'nervous energy,' and when I read that it is the basis of life, I confess that this conveys no meaning to me. Perhaps Prof. Rignano means to speak of 'psychic energy,' of Spirit or of the Soul? If so, that is quite another matter, and it does not appear to me suitable to call Spirit 'nervous energy.' It may be that Spirit is the basis of life, but in that case it is also the basis of every natural event in the inorganic world both of universal gravitation and of the simplest chemical equilibrium, as well as of every affective tendency whatever, animal or human. We may, if we wish to do so, adopt the language of physics and call Spirit 'energy,' but on condition

that we at once make clear that in so doing we over-
step the bounds of dynamical science, because we
do not yet know from what other forms of energy
Spirit can arise, or into what others it can be changed
in accordance with dynamical principles. Perhaps,
on the other hand, Prof. Rignano merely means the
specific functional activity of nervous tissue as other
authors speak of 'muscular energy' or 'secretory
energy.' This, however, seems to me inadmissible.
Sponges live and exhibit movements of their sphincters without possessing a trace of nervous tissue;
how then can nervous energy be the basis of their
life?

"In spite of the researches of Brailsford Robertson
and others, we do not know what is the physiological
basis of the mnemonic faculty or of the power of
accumulation, not only in the most sharply defined
form of this faculty which is peculiar to nervous
tissue, but even of the more obscure and rudimentary
form of it, which, since Hering, many assume to
belong to living matter in general. We do not know
what it is that accumulates, or what the 'traces'
are which are accumulated, of which many speak
so confidently, contenting themselves thus with a
phrase devoid of concrete meaning. One thing,
however, is certain, and that is that since Van
Bemmelen, physical chemists recognise in non-living
colloidal systems well-defined mnemonic properties.
It therefore seems to me that we cannot consider
these properties as characteristic of living organised
systems only, and that to attempt to explain the
affective tendencies by the mnemonic properties of

BIOLOGICAL MEMORY

protoplasm is to put forward an explanation of one unknown by another unknown.

"Let us, however, get to the heart of Prof. Rignano's address, to the question of the purposefulness or finalism of vital phenomena. If instead of ' the tendency to stability' (invariance), Prof. Rignano had spoken of the ' tendency to the preservation of equilibrium,' he would have given a more correct expression of the matter. It is indeed permissible to doubt whether the concept of ' stability ' is applicable to living organisms at all. What these organisms strive to maintain is not *a given equilibrium*, which would be equivalent to immobility, but just *equilibrium in general* under different conditions of the environment. When an animal has satisfied its hunger, or adapted itself to a temperature very different from that to which it had become accustomed, equilibrium is restored within its body, but this is a new equilibrium implying different internal conditions, which are either apparent or are not appreciable with our means of observation. The animal which to-day has satisfied its hunger is really different from the same animal when it assuaged its hunger yesterday, as Leonardo da Vinci has already pointed out, just as the animal which has become adapted to a higher temperature is different, but in this case to a much greater extent, from the same animal before the adaptation has taken place.

"Now, I do not see any essential difference in this respect between living systems and inorganic systems, since the tendency to the preservation of equilibrium is equally characteristic of both. In a system composed of carbonate of calcium, of oxide of calcium, and of carbon dioxide, there will always exist a definite state of equilibrium at every temperature and under every degree of pressure ; this equilibrium when disturbed will be restored each time in a different way ; and to each state of equilibrium there will correspond different internal conditions, because the masses of the two solid components of the system will change and also the pressure or molecular concentration of the gaseous component. And one could speak of this inorganic system as displaying purpose as justly as Messrs. Jennings and Rignano speak of the living organism.

" A similar but much more complex case is that of the preservation of the equilibrium between the hydrogen ions and the hydroxyl ions of the blood, which constitutes the normal reaction of this liquid. To every increase in the partial pressure of CO_2 the system responds by a corresponding fixation of this gas effected by the available bases. But if the pressure exceed a certain limit, it produces a reaction of the protoplasm of certain nerve-cells situated in the spinal bulb (respiratory centre) which then send out stimuli to the respiratory muscles, the rhythm of respiration is accelerated, and the respiration become deeper, and the excess of CO_2 is thus got rid of and so equilibrium is re-established in the blood. Let us picture to ourselves a vessel containing the same inorganic system as we have just described, and provided with a valve which will open and allow the excess of CO_2 to escape when the pressure of this gas exceeds a certain limit. I can heat this system, that is, cause the decomposition of $CaCO_3$, and the increase of the concentration of CO_2 in the space above the solid, but the normal pressure of the gas, that is, the condition of equilibrium, will always eventually be restored, granted the presence of the valve which will allow of the escape of the excess of CO_2. Shall we say that ' this system seems to strive to attain a definite end,' that ' the final result of its activity seems in some way to be present from the beginning, governing what the action shall be,' and that ' the final result of its action is effectively present from the beginning under the form of a mnemonic accumulation constituting a *vis a fronte* or *final cause* ' ?

" I could, of course, continue this argument, but I prefer to conclude by a short general discussion of the matter.

" What is really important is to learn to know and to explain natural phenomena, those of psychic life as well as those of vegetable and animal life, and those which are manifested by non-living systems ; and it seems to me that in describing them we should abstain from attributing to them our ideas of purpose which are a peculiar habit of our minds. To mingle these human ideas with natural phenomena by attributing purpose to the latter, seems to me, to say the least of it, an arbitrary proceeding and may even be dangerous.

" There was a time when in physics and chemistry we habitually made use of a language implying purpose (fire strives to reach the sky, nature abhors a vacuum, oxygen has tendency to unite with hydrogen). Now this language has either disappeared or persists only as an out-of-date livery covering well defined concepts. At the time of which we speak, the differences between the description of vital phenomena and those of the inorganic world were less acute than they are at present. A time will soon come, or at least we hope so, when language like that used by Prof. Jennings and Prof. Rignano will also have disappeared from physiology, and when the difference between the descriptions of physiological phenomena and those of physics and chemistry will again have become less obvious, by a change in the opposite direction, the former becoming as fundamentally and essentially objective as the second are at present, without any admixture of ' final causes,' of ' affective tendencies ' and of ' menmonic accumulations,' which are at present mere forms of words since they refer to observed facts of the nature of which we are ignorant and of the effective causes of which we know nothing. Now in natural science it is not permissible—for it would lead to very serious consequences—to work with verbal expressions denoting facts and phenomena of unknown nature, because, if we do so, we run the risk of confounding causes with effects, of mistaking superficial analogies with profound causal relations, of substituting pretences of explanation for real explanation, thus perpetuating and increasing a confusion of ideas which is certainly not calculated to promote the progress of science towards the discovery of truth."

CHAPTER XI

PHYSICO - CHEMICAL THEORIES AND MNEMONIC
THEORIES CONSIDERED IN RELATION TO THE
MOST CHARACTERISTIC MANIFESTATIONS OF LIFE.
THE MNEMONIC POINT OF VIEW

To refuse to attribute any value to conceptions or hypotheses which cannot be immediately tested by experiment is too narrow a standpoint for any scientist to adopt. The mechanists confound essentially different things when they assert that inorganic systems manifest mnemonic properties. It is not the mere capacity for adaptation, that is to say, the capacity of continually establishing a state of equilibrium with the forces of the external world, but the tendency to reproduce a pre-determined adaptation, the longing for the old environment, the struggle towards a definite end, which constitute the essential differences between physico-chemical systems and organisms. Prof. Bottazzi's vessel containing a non-living mixture of materials developing a gas and provided with a valve, is a *machine*, and as such it is a purposeful (finalistic) manifestation of the human mind. It is the very technique of the physicists and chemists applied to organic phenomena which prevents the recognition of the various purposeful manifestations of life—ontogenetic, morphological, instinctive and affective—but these purposeful manifestations are nevertheless *facts*. This limitation of outlook on the part of the thorough specialist emphasises the necessity of collaboration between the synthetical theorist and the experimental specialist.

THE criticisms which the eminent physiologist of the University of Naples has levelled at my study of the purposefulness of life show quite clearly, not only the value, but the necessity of that collaboration between the synthetic theorists, and the experimental specialists, which has long been established in the realm of the physical sciences where laboratory researches and mathematical speculation render to one another continual and reciprocal aid, but which is almost completely wanting in the realm of the biological science.

If the pure scientists reply to the too narrow views of those who desire to see immediately the practical results of every theoretical speculation by showing the enormous injury which would be done to science by this too utilitarian outlook, it is but just to make a similar objection to the attitude of those extreme specialists who are inclined to deny all value to conceptions and hypotheses which cannot be immediately tested experimentally. For indeed certain general conceptions, even if it is impossible to submit them at once to the test of experiment, may nevertheless be of great value in allowing of a comprehensive view of a confused mass of phenomena, which till now have seemed to be totally unrelated to one another, and in thus providing a platform from which it is possible to plan future researches. Hypotheses, which as yet cannot be tested experimentally, may be amenable to experiment in the near future, just as certain theories of pure science which have remained without practical applications, even for centuries, have finally received such applications, often of great utility. Finally, synthetic views may very well serve to remind specialists, too prone to be satisfied with their results, that certain categories of phenomena, including some of quite fundamental importance, still await an explanation to which the path followed by the specialists has not, and cannot, bring us a step nearer.

Thus our critic says that he knows nothing of nervous energy, and that the term conveys no meaning to him. Now it is true that no one has yet proved the existence of this energy by experiments in the laboratory, but it is a conception easily comprehensible by the student of dynamics that there should be a form of energy which, although it faithfully obeys the general laws of energetics, manifests properties peculiar to itself and found in no other form of energy ¬met with in the inorganic world. If then the hypothesis of the existence of a new form of energy, endowed with well-defined properties peculiar to itself, allows us to take a more comprehensive view of all the phenomena of life and to distinguish them sharply from inorganic phenomena, in opposition to the tendency of physiological specialists to consider both categories to be of the same nature—a tendency due to the technique employed by them by which both living and non-living matter are subjected to the same physico-chemical treatment—then we can see the value of this conception of such a nervous energy, even if the existence of this energy has not yet been experimentally demonstrated.

The conception of such a form of energy, obeying the general laws of energetics, but endowed with properties peculiar to itself, possessed by no other form of inorganic energy, is not in any way anti-scientific, nor does it involve any metaphysics, and it has especially nothing to do with the old metaphysical conception of the soul and I am astonished that my critic has not recognised the abyss which divides these two conceptions.

" Sponges," says our critic, " live and manifest movements of their muscular sphincters without possessing a trace of nervous tissue ; how then can nervous energy be the basis of their life ? " In making this statement M. Bottazzi has evidently forgotten the fundamental conception of Claude Bernard as to the essential identity of the nature of all the various forms of irritability of living substance. For it is in entire conformity with Bernard's views if we assume that the same energy, which constitutes the irritability of nervous substance, is the basis of every other kind of irritability of living matter, and that the different varieties of the various nuclear discharges of a single form of energy give rise in protoplasm to various physico-chemical phenomena, which manifest themselves as different physiological actions (such as muscular contraction and glandular secretion and so on). Without the aid of Bernard's conception of the essential identity of all the various forms of irritability of living substance, we should have difficulty in assuming that evolution had really occurred, for we should be unable to understand how nervous energy, if it is only the specific functional activity of a single tissue, could have appeared in animals now possessing this tissue, but descended from ancestors which were devoid of such a tissue. Nor could we understand ontogenetic development if we did not assume the existence, even in the fertilised egg and in the blastula and gastrula stages, of the same energy which later manifests itself in a more striking manner in the nervous tissues of the adult. There is certainly no need for me to remind M. Bottazzi how the lower

organisms devoid of this tissue and even the unicellular animals show, by their behaviour, certain
preferences, make choices, and in certain cases give
indubitable evidence of having profited by past
experience, all phenomena which in higher animals
are attributed to the functional activity of nervous
tissue.

" We are completely ignorant," writes Prof.
Bottazzi " of the physiological basis of the mnemonic
faculty." We agree on this point and we likewise
agree that the hypothesis of the property of forming
specific accumulations—a property which distinguishes nervous energy from all the other forms
of energy in the inorganic world—is as yet not
capable of being verified experimentally. But, apart
from any hypothesis, we have given a definition of
biological memory, which only expresses in a general
formula the facts which everyone regards as manifestations of this mnemonic property of living matter.
We have, in fact, defined it as the property of
reproducing by the action of internal causes given
physiological states for the original production of
which external causes were necessary. We may
know nothing of the nature of these internal causes,
but we recognise a series of varied phenomena which
can all be compressed within this definition. We
observe, for instance, that the secretion of certain
gastric juices produced at first in a herbivorous
animal through its being gradually accustomed to a
diet of flesh, is subsequently reproduced by internal
causes, that is, it is no longer produced merely as a
consequence of what is swallowed, but by the mere

perception of the smell of this kind of food. Similarly we observe that certain new rhythms (of the opening and shutting up of leaves, of the increase and the diminution of the turgescence produced by the sap, and so on) acquired by a plant as a consequence of the alternation of artificial light and darkness differing in period from those of day and night, persist for some time without modification whether the plant be exposed to continuous illumination or to continuous darkness, or again to natural daylight. We associate these phenomena on the one hand with the fact that the sight of a given panorama which represents a momentary physiological state of our brains, can be subsequently exactly reproduced as a memory, that is to say in the absence of the external agent ; and we associate them on the other hand with the development of the embryo itself which reproduces by the action of internal causes given physiological and morphological states, which undoubtedly must have owed their origin in previous generations to functional adaptations, that is to the action of definite external agents.

If the natural inorganic world—excluding certain machines manufactured for this purpose by man, such as the phonograph and others like it—contained physico-chemical systems which possessed the property that certain of their dynamical states produced in the first instance by the surrounding world and ceasing to exist as such when the environment became modified, could be subsequently reproduced without the action of the same environment, then we could really assert that the mnemonic property was not peculiar to life, but belonged also to the inorganic world.

But we see that it is impossible to include in this category either the lasting of the impressions or deformations which solid bodies undergo by the action of given external pressures, or the hysteresis manifested by iron in a variable field of magnetic force, or the traces which colloidal systems retain of all the modifications to which they have been subjected, or other similar phenomena often adduced as instances of inorganic memory, and all due simply to the persistence of definite effects after the causes which produced them have ceased to operate.

In other words memory is not " any after-effect of external causes," as it is defined by Loeb and those who, like him, wish to give the word as wide an embrace as that of the Divine Mercy, but rather the reproduction of dynamical effects without the renewed aid of the corresponding external conditions *and after the effects due to these conditions have completely ceased to exist.* In this sense the mnemonic property belongs exclusively and peculiarly to life.

Our critic asserts that to try to explain the affective tendencies by the mnemonic property is to attempt to explain one unknown by another unknown. On this point we must take note of the meaning which positive philosophy assigns to the word " explain." Since the time of Comte, and indeed since the ancient Greek philosophers, when we succeed in associating together as similar, phenomena which had previously appeared entirely different, that in itself is an explanation.

Now we have striven to show that all the principal organic affective tendencies, however different from each other they seem to us, can all be comprised in the one single tendency of the organism to maintain its physiological stability, a tendency of which the different affective tendencies are individual manifestations. We can, of course, seek for an explanation of this fundamental tendency which includes all the others, but even if this were actually inexplicable, the fact that we had been able to include all the other tendencies within it would, none the less, be an explanation of these.

But we have endeavoured in turn to compare this unique comprehensive tendency with other needs or desires of animals in general and of men in particular, which have arisen through the action of habit, and thus we have referred all the affective tendencies, both inborn and acquired, to the mnemonic property as we have defined it above. Since, moreover, we had already in previous studies also referred other purposeful phenomena of life, and amongst them the most fundamental of all, to this mnemonic property— from the perfect pre-adaptation of each organism to its environment and from ontogenetic development, which forms organs not called on to exercise their functions until the adult stage is reached, on the one hand, to the complex instincts of animals, which provide in advance for their future needs, down to simple reflex acts, already so perfectly " mechanised " for the preservation and well being of the organism, on the other hand—we have a perfect right to say that we have " explained " all the purposeful manifestations of life by referring them to the unique phenomenon of *mnemonic reproduction*. This phenomenon, let us repeat, we can content ourselves by defining as the reproduction by internal causes of morphogenetic and physiological phenomena, which were in the first instance produced by the action of external agents.

This grouping of all purposeful manifestations of life under one head is, in itself, a real explanation of them, *even if we were completely ignorant of the inner mechanism of this mnemonic property*, which, however, we have tried to explain by the theory of specific accumulations, characteristic of that nervous energy which we have assumed to be the basis of all vital phenomena, so that our critic does not do us justice in affirming that we have explained nothing at all.

But let us go on, as our critic demands, to what he calls the heart of the matter, to the points which embody the real diversity between our theoretical views. M. Bottazzi seems not to perceive the radical difference between the simple tendency to establish equilibrium with changing external conditions, that is to say to become adapted to them and the tendency to preserve or to restore, after it is disturbed, a given condition of equilibrium, attained in a definite environment which has remained unchanged for some time.

" The animal which has satisfied its hunger to-day," says M. Bottazzi, "is different from the same animal which has assuaged its hunger yesterday, just as the animal which has become adapted to a higher temperature is different from the same animal before the adaptation has occurred." No, we reply, the two cases are entirely different : the animal which has satisfied its hunger has by so doing succeeded in restoring its normal physiological condition, and that is why it no longer experiences any desire to eat ; on the contrary, the animal placed in a medium of a higher temperature than that to which it is accustomed, will at first make every possible effort to return to conditions of normal temperature, and thus to restore its former physiological state which has been disturbed ; and it is only after all its efforts have failed, that it will establish itself in a new state of physiological equilibrium with the modified environment. The animal will retain for a certain time a " longing " for the old environment, which will still allow of its reviving the old state of physiological equilibrium now reduced to a potential condition, and it is only after a much longer period that this longing will give place to an " affectivity " (attachment) towards this new environment ; this change will occur when the new physiological state has had time to deposit a sufficient quantity of mnemonic accumulation to give rise to the new affectivity.

As far as the faculty of adaptation is concerned, by which is meant the power of continually reaching a condition of equilibrium with external forces, I agree with Prof. Bottazzi, as I have indeed expressly admitted in the preceding chapter on " Teleologism and Memory," that there appears to be in this respect no essential difference between living and inorganic systems, since this power of ever anew reaching a state of equilibrium with the environment is a general property of energy, shared by all the forms of energy. What constitutes the difference between physico-chemical systems and organisms, is the *longing for the old environment.* This longing can be observed in organisms even as low as the protista, as is shown by their negative reaction to the new environment and their positive reaction to the old one, a behaviour so brilliantly observed and described by Jennings. Consequently the instances cited by Prof. Bottazzi of the tendency, also of inorganic systems, to reach a condition of equilibrium with the environment are irrelevant, because none of these inorganic systems exhibit anything similar to such a " longing."

For instance his system, composed of calcium, oxide of calcium and carbon dioxide, which reaches a new condition of equilibrium when the temperature changes, shows no tendency to persist in its previous temperature, whilst Paramecium reacts negatively to every rise or fall of temperature however slight, just as Euglena reacts negatively to every change in the intensity of the illumination of the medium to which it has become accustomed.

But it is Prof. Bottazzi himself who provides us with an argument against his own thesis, in the example which he cites, of the reaction of the organism to too high a pressure of carbon dioxide in the blood ; for whilst a physico-chemical system would simply reach a new state of equilibrium with the higher degree of pressure, the organism on the contrary reacts by stimuli transmitted to the respiratory muscles by an accelerated rhythm of respirations and by deeper respirations, *so as to expel the excess of carbon dioxide and thus to re-establish in the blood the normal condition of equilibrium which had been disturbed.*

But, replies M. Bottazzi, this reaction may be compared to what would happen if we heated a system, like that described above, composed of carbonate of calcium, oxide of calcium, and carbon dioxide, *if we imagine that the vessel in which it is contained was provided with a valve which would open and allow CO_2 to escape when the pressure of this gas exceeded a certain limit.*

It seems to have completely escaped M. Bottazzi's notice, that this valve planned and placed in position precisely in order to prevent the pressure of carbon dioxide exceeding a certain limit, *is in itself a phenomenon which is a purposeful manifestation of the human mind.* Therefore the system, which he describes is indeed an inorganic system, but one which has been pre-arranged by man in order to attain certain ends, and it is only for this reason that it can be compared in certain respects to the purposefulness shown by organic systems. In other words, the system postulated by Prof. Bottazzi is a *machine,* and like all other machines, it bears the characteristic imprint of the purposefulness of man, an imprint which can never be found in *natural* inorganic systems. The comparison, which he institutes between our respiratory system, which tends to maintain invariable the pressure of carbon dioxide gas in the blood, and a machine, only brings into stronger relief the purposeful character of the respiratory system.

Let us now deal with the general considerations

with which Prof. Bottazzi concludes his criticism. "What is really important," he writes, "is to learn to know and to explain natural phenomena, those of psychic life as well as those of animal and vegetable life, and those which are manifested in non-living systems, and it seems to me that in describing them we should abstain from attributing to them our ideas of purpose, *which are a peculiar habit to our minds.*" Now I ask, is not this habit of the human mind also a phenomenon pertaining to life ? By the phrase which I have underlined does not M. Bottazzi himself *admit the essentially purposeful character which our minds at least possess ?* Moreover, this purposeful habit is not a property belonging peculiarly and exclusively to our minds, since all the behaviour of animals from the higher organisms most nearly allied to us, down to the very lowest, appears to be quite comparable with our own purposeful behaviour, but even if such a " finalistic " habit were limited to our minds, it would constitute a perfect valid purposefulness of life, the existence of which is thus conceded by our critic.

The ancient anthropomorphic tendency to see man in everything, or at least behaviours analogous to those of man, has been succeeded by the opposite and not less dangerous tendency, due entirely to the fault of the laboratory specialists, *to forget man*, that is to say, to forget that man with all his needs, affectivities and aspirations, exists and is *a fact* not less real than the precipitation of a salt or the coagulation of a colloid.

It is true that the biochemists have never had the opportunity of seeing in their retorts any manifestation of affectivity, or other purposeful manifestation of life, because the purposeful nature of certain vital phenomena *only becomes apparent in the relation between actual phenomena and certain future phenomena, separated from each other by a certain interval of time,* as, for instance, between the formation of the baby's eye in the darkness of the mother's womb, and its future use when it will be exposed to the light of the outer world, between the present behaviour of the swallow which builds its nest and the future use of the nest when the same swallow will lay its eggs in it, between the present act of a man who is making a machine and the future use that he will make of the machine. The biochemist only observes the mutual relations of phenomena which immediately succeed one another. It follows that, in virtue of his technique, he never has the opportunity of observing purposeful phenomena, and therefore he denies their existence, just as the colour-blind man is tempted to deny the existence of certain colours. Sooner than admit the utter incapacity of his technique to study, or to explain the purposeful manifestations of life, the biochemist gets rid of the question by simply denying the existence of these manifestations *which are nevertheless facts.*

Further, this technique which brings him into close contact with, and teaches him to know the fully formed organism, is not the most suitable to keep constantly before his mind the consideration that the phenomenal relations which his technique enables him gradually to discover, as due to the mode of working of the machine which is the organism, even if they were entirely explicable by the mode of being of that machine, confront us with the most fundamental problem of all to solve, viz., to explain *how the machine succeds in the course of ontogeny in constructing itself.* Thus, to take the example of the respiratory mechanism cited above, when the physiologist has discovered that the increase in the pressure of carbon dioxide gas evokes a reaction in the protoplasm of certain nerve cells situated in the spinal bulb which thereupon emit stimuli to the respiratory muscles, he imagines that he has explained the phenomenon of the constancy of the pressure of carbon dioxide in the blood, and he does not perceive that the still more important phenomenon which remains to be explained, is the *existence of the mechanism so well adapted to accomplish this end.*

The fact that manifestations of purpose are exclusively peculiar to life, naturally made sterile the explanations of inorganic phenomena by phrases implying purpose (as the fire striving to reach the sky, nature abhorring a vacuum, the sympathy of oxygen for hydrogen and so on), but for the very same reasons it also renders sterile each attempt to explain the living world by means of physico-chemical expressions.

This impotence of physics and chemistry to explain the purposefulness of life, becomes naturally more obvious as we approach the phenomena of the true psychic life, in which the signs of purposefulness appear with more brilliant clearness.

It is at this point that some physiologists, and amongst them our critic, are driven into a corner and take refuge in spiritualism ; that is to say they distinguish sharply between psychical and physio-- logical phenomena. For instance, Bottazzi expresses himself thus :   " In my opinion physiological phenomena, *amongst which I do not reckon psychic phenomena,* are, or will be, capable of being causally explained, just like the phenomena of the inorganic world. Since both are actual processes we cannot admit that there is any essential difference between them. I can only discover a difference, and that an essential one, between physical and physiological phenomena, on the one hand, and psychic or spiritual phenomena on the other. Thus I believe it possible to be at the same time a spiritualist in philosophy, and a non-vitalist and to deny any purpose in phy- siology." It is in these words that Prof. Bottazzi writes to me in the course of a private and courteous discussion which has preceded this public discussion.

Now I ask if this admission is not a clear proof of the danger to which extreme specialism is exposed of erecting impassable barriers between sciences which are in many ways allied, and that not on account of the inner nature of the phenomena studied, but on account of the similar or dissimilar technique employed in the study of them. This procedure makes clear the necessity of a synthetic outlook which, overriding the limitations of any given technique, will enable us to grasp the essential characteristics of phenomena and to unite them in a single view, thus restoring to unity sciences which have been artifically separated by different methods of technique.

Is it indeed possible, we may ask, for anyone who

views the multitudinous complexity of organic phenomena as a whole to distinguish sharply between physiological and psychological phenomena ? In which category are we to place hunger and the other fundamental organic needs and the sexual instinct itself, which I have discussed in detail in the chapter on the purposefulness of life ? Do they not rather constitute the bridge which connects the two categories of phenomena, and by which the one variety passes into the other ? Are they to be considered psychical phenomena in man, especially when they are transformed into more complex and more elevated affectivities, and as physiological phenomena in animals in whom they manifest themselves by acts of ferocity, by sexual combats and so on ? Should the flight of a frightened child be considered as a purely psychic phenomenon, whilst that of a dog at the sight of its master's whip, or the efforts of an amœba to escape from the interior of another amœba, so beautifully described by Jennings, should these phenomena, on the other hand, be considered purely physiological ? Shall we reckon as purely physiological the instinct of the ant which carries provision for the winter into its subterranean abode, whilst we regard as purely psychological the action of the poor old woman who laboriously collects and carries off the dry branches which she has found by the way-side in order to make a good blaze ? All these are questions, which not only is the specialist unable to answer, but which never occur to his mind, just because, I repeat, he does not encounter them in his particular laboratory researches, but they continally tantalise and puzzle the synthetic theorist. The theorist might also be permitted to say that the real fundamental questions are precisely those which the specialist either does not see or which he neglects, and that the most intimately connected problems are just those which the specialist divides between distinct sciences, artificially sharply separated from one another.

In view of these circumstances the synthetic theorist succeeds, at least, in proving the absolute necessity of synthesis for the real progress of science, which must consist, let us not forget, not in the chaotic amassing of minute facts, but in the comprehensive insight into their numerous mutual relations.

I am, however, most grateful to my friend, the illustrious physiologist, for his detailed and penetrating criticisms, which have enabled me to state more clearly my conceptions of biological synthesis.

After having thus set forth and defended the explanation of the purposeful or finalistic manifestations *of life* which is provided by the mnemonic theory, it remains to be shown that this theory is also capable of accounting for the equally purposeful phenomena *of the mind*. It is only when this task has been accomplished that we shall be able to state that we have really acquired a comprehensive unitary view of both life and mind. It is to this task that we shall devote ourselves in the two following chapters with which this work will conclude.

CHAPTER XII

BIOLOGICAL MEMORY AND THE FUNCTIONING OF THE INTELLIGENCE[1]

Analysis and synthesis of our intelligence. Biological memory is able to account for the elements of which the intelligence is composed. The "affective tendencies." The emotions. The will. Attention. Reason. Coherence and logic. Advantages and disadvantages of reasoning compared with those of actual experiment. The ground of the fertility of reasoning as an instrument of research.

WHEN the psychologist undertakes to study such a difficult problem as the functioning of the intelligence, it is absolutely necessary that he should see clearly that his task is, first, the preliminary work of analysing the more complex psychic phenomena into less complex ones, and these in turn into others still more elementary, until he arrives at the most elementary phenomena of all, by the composition of which all other psychic phenomena are formed, and secondly, synthetic work in which, starting from these elements, he endeavours to show how all the most complex manifestations of intellect are built up. This is what I have attempted to do in my work entitled " The Psychology of Reasoning." In this work, beginning with the most complex psychic phenomenon of all, which is reasoning, we proceed with our analysis until

[1] A paper communicated to the Congress of the American, English, French and Italian Philosophical Societies held in Paris from the 27th to the 31st of December, 1921.

we reach the two most elementary psychic phenomena, which resist further psychological analysis, viz., first, the elementary "affective tendencies," and secondly, sensations and memories of sensations, and then we show how from the combination of these phenomena all the intellectual functions and faculties are derived.

THE AFFECTIVE TENDENCIES

Whilst sensations and the corresponding memories of sensations have been fully studied in their different aspects by an army of philosophers, psychologists, physiologists and anatomists, the study of the affective tendencies (not to be confounded with the emotions), on the contrary, has until now been almost completely neglected, probably because the majority of observers have failed to notice the supreme importance of these tendencies in all manifestations of thought ; and it is the manifestations of thought alone which formerly interested scientific researchers. It is only quite recently and almost exclusively in the domain of psychiatry, that interest in the affective tendencies has been awakened, and Ribot is the first who has begun, though somewhat obscurely, to catch a glimpse of the large part which they play in all the processes of the psychic life, even in those that are most elevated and most complex.

It has, therefore, seemed necessary to us to enquire with more care than has hitherto been employed in the task, what are the origin, nature, and most fundamental properties of these affective tendencies, in order better to understand the different ways in which they enter into and help to build up the highest faculties of reason. This is, indeed, what we have done in the first chapter of our work alluded to above, and in the address on " The Purposefulness of Life," which we had the honour to deliver in Paris to the College of France, and which we have reproduced in Chapters VIII and IX of this book.

In these studies, in which we started with the lowest organisms and then proceeded upwards till we reached man, we demonstrated the existence of three groups of affective tendencies. Those of the first group, such as hunger, thirst, the tendency to maintain unchanged its own environment, the need of getting rid of various substances which are either useless or noxious to the organism, the sexual instinct itself, in which is manifested the desire to get rid of the germinal substance and of the disturbance caused by it, and other similar organic " desires," " appetites " or " needs," are only so many different forms of the characteristic tendency of the organism to uphold its physiological stability, that is, to retain its normal physiological state unchanged, and to restore this state when it has been disturbed.

The second group comprises all those needs, appetites and desires which arise as the result of habit, and in this category we placed, for instance, the intense desire which arises for certain relations of symbiosis or parastism, such as those of mother and child, when these relations have lasted for a considerable time ; from such a relation maternal love has arisen and been developed ; and in the same category belong family affections in general, friendship and other social relations, and all the needs acquired in life by every customary relation to the environment, and finally all the most varied " longings " (" nostalgias ") and regrets.

The third group consists of the derivative and composite affective tendencies which have arisen from the affective tendencies of the two preceding groups, either by way of " affective transference " (from the whole to the part, from the end to the means, from one element of the environment to another which is its concomitant, from an object to an analogous one: law of transference of Ribot) or by way of the combination of two or more affective tendencies which enter simultaneously into action. Such component tendencies either coalesce completely, or one partially modifies or inhibits another, thus giving rise to a unique complex resultant, which according to the number, quality and intensity of its components, may constitute any one of the infinite number of nuances of which human feelings are capable.

Further we have succeeded in showing that all these three groups can be derived from that peculiar property of mnemonic accumulation which, in our opinion, is the fundamental property of living matter; so that it appeared to us that the awakening (activation) of an affective tendency is a kind of mnemonic revival, but with properties which are only partially analogous to those of sensory memories and which are partly peculiar to itself. These peculiar properties are due to the fact of the primitive visceral origin of all the most fundamental organic affective tendencies, which constitute the real foundation of all the affective edifice of the psyché.

Our task is now to show how from this stock of affective tendencies, on the one hand, and of sensations or revivals of sensations on the other, there originate and develop all the operations of the intelligence and the highest manifestations of thought.

THE EMOTIONS, THE WILL, AND THE ATTENTION.

We must begin by making a distinction, almost always neglected by the majority of psychologists, between the affective tendencies and the emotions. These latter are only sudden and intense discharges of the energy which constitutes the affective tendencies. Each affective tendency, which becomes active, strives towards movement, that is to say, it presses on (" impinges on " in Sherrington's words) the corresponding locomotor organs, and thus reveals itself from the moment of its awakening as a nascent movement. If, however, the tendency is excited in a sudden and intense fashion, there is a great outpouring of nervous energy, which being suddenly released in great quantity inundates the organism and floods, not only the path connected with the locomotor apparatus, but many others as well, giving rise to a visceral commotion which, according to the well-known theory of James, Lange and Sergi, reverberates afterwards in the brain under the guise of an emotion. If, on the contrary, the awakening of the affective tendency is neither sudden nor too intense, it results only in the stimulation of the necessary muscles, without any emotion, and it yields an output of useful work which is greater in proportion to the smaller quantity of the discharge which is wasted in the disorderly and useless visceral disturbance which only produces emotion.

As regards the will, we have an act of volition every time that an " affective tendency," directed towards a future end, is successful in overcoming an affective tendency seeking immediate satisfaction. Thus, when a man, breathless and bathed in perspiration as the result of a long race, throws himself greedily on the first spring of water which he finds and begins to drink, he is not performing an act of will, but such an act is performed by a man who abstains from satisfying his burning thirst from fear of the future damage to himself which might result from this satisfaction. It is not an act of will when a tired man throws himself down on the ground to rest, but it is such an act when an Alpinist overcomes his fatigue in order to reach the peak which he is striving to climb. The will is therefore in essence only an affective tendency of wider vision and one which inhibits other tendencies which aim at more immediate satisfaction ; that is why it excites to action like every other affective tendency.

Attention is similar to the will in some respects and different from it in others ; like the will it is the result of a conflict of affective tendencies, but the conflict occurs between a primary affective tendency which seeks a definite good, and a secondary tendency which inhibits for some time the primary one, from the fear that, by allowing the primary one to become active too soon, this tendency will not succeed in attaining the desired end. Thus, the savage animal which sees its prey approaching it in ignorance of danger, does not at once spring upon its victim, but, though excited by the most ardent desire, waits motionless, with all the muscles which will be used in the future spring in tension, until the poor animal approaches still nearer and comes within its reach. Likewise the scientific man, who is observing through a microscope or telescope, " with great attention," a given object, is moved by the desire to see a phenomenon which will constitute a final proof of his theories, or which will be a great discovery, and he is at the same time obsessed with the fear, when he believes that he sees what he is looking for, lest he should be the victim of an optical illusion, and it is this fear which prevents him from concluding too hastily that he has really seen the desired thing.

As a result of the effect which affective tendencies have in reviving sensations and images when these are in accordance with their aims, and in enfeebling and inhibiting sensations and images opposed to them, the fact that the object, observed or considered " with attention," is subjected to two affective points of view at the same time, evidently results in a greater exactitude of perception or recollection. We might express this metaphorically by saying that the object becomes thus exposed, not to one, but to two beams of light from two internal reflectors, which illuminate it on several sides at once. The effect of this is to bring into relief a whole series of properties which would never have been noticed if only a single affectivity had come into action. For this reason attentive observation yields much more exact and precise results than that made under the influence of a single affectivity, whilst observation guided by a single affective point of view, especially if the affectivity is too intense, may yield erroneous results quite divergent from reality.

REASONING

If we examine and analyse concrete examples of reasoning selected from amongst the most simple and familiar ones, or from amongst those, for instance, employed to solve certain riddles like the classical one of the shepherd, the wolf, the goat, and the cabbage, or from amongst those met with in elementary mathematics like the proof that the sum of the angles of a triangle is equal to two right angles and other similar problems, reasoning will appear to us to be nothing more than *a series of inter-connected experiments conceived, but not actually performed.* In other words, it is made up of experiments on a given object of special interest to ourselves, which we perform in imagination but do not really carry out, because from the results of similar experiments actually carried out in the past, we know beforehand what the result of each separate experiment will be. The final experimental result mentally " observed " or " determined," to which this series or chain of merely imagined experiments leads up, is in point of fact " the result of the demonstration " or " the conclusion of the reasoning." Thus, for instance, when we follow " with the eyes of the mind " the merely imagined transportation of a simple pendulum from a cold to a warm room, we observe or verify in our minds, by our memories of experiments actually performed in the past on the effect of heat on metallic rods, that the pendulum will increase in length ; and by recalling other experiments also previously performed, we then determine mentally that the pendulum will swing more slowly than before.

Thus we find in this case that a combination of two imagined experiments and the act of connecting the two corresponding successive mental observations or determinations, of which the second constitutes the conclusion of this short and simple piece of reasoning, enable us to know that the transportation of a pendulum from a cold to a warm medium will slow down the clockwork, the speed of which is regulated by the pendulum.

The person who in reasoning thinks "with attention" is primarily governed by an affective tendency, which by means of the revival of suitable sensory memories imagines and follows the different combinations of experiments which he mentally performs on an object, which at the moment arouses his particular interest. In a word the individual, who is reasoning, follows the imagined vicissitudes of the object about which he is thinking, in the same fashion, and with the same interest, as the hunter follows with his glances the movements, disappearances, concealments, reappearances and other vicissitudes of the prey which he desires to possess. It is this primary affective tendency, always active throughout the whole course of the reasoning, which constitutes the psychic constant which connects together the imagined experiments to which the object, which interests the reasoning individual, is subjected. It is the greater or less capacity of persistence of this affective tendency on which depends *the coherence or incoherence* of the whole intellectual process when this requires a considerable time to reach its complete development.

The secondary affective tendency, which at each step in attentive reasoning holds the primary tendency in check, is the fear of attributing to each imagined experiment a result which would not be exactly the same as would be obtained if the experiment were actually carried out. Under the stimulus of this fear, an increasing number of more or less similar past experiments are recalled to the memory, and indeed by preference those which give antagonistic results to those which might have been thought of at first under the influence of the primary desire that the result might be in one direction rather than in another. It is, therefore, the continual control exercised by the secondary affective tendency to which is due *the logic* of reasoning, since logic consists only in assigning to every imagined experiment the result which it would really give if it were actually carried out.

Insane people with their want of "mental balance"—which is nothing but want of affective equilibrium—and their extravagant reasoning which results from it, provide a confirmation of the different parts played in reasoning by the primary and secondary affectivities. There is, indeed, a whole category of insane people, the paranoiacs, who, although they manifest the greatest *coherence* as a consequence of the very great persistence of the single affectivity, which being always active in them forms the kernel around which their monomania revolves, nevertheless exhibit the greatest want of *logic*. This is due to the fact that in them the intensity of their primary affective tendency is so great that no secondary affective tendency can arise which is capable of checking the primary one, even for an instant ; as a consequence, all the results obtained by paranoiacs from their mental experiments are consonant, not with reality, but with what their single affective tendency desires or fears. On the other hand in *maniacs*, who show the greatest affective instability and variability, in *the confused cases*, in whom the paths by which the affective tendencies exercise their action of revival, selection and inhibition of the sensory memories, are blocked, and finally in *the déments*, in whom all awakening of affectivities is lacking, it is *incoherence* which constitutes the most typical manifestation of their psyché. Moreover, in *dreams*, even in those of the normal man, in which the subsidence of the affectivities which is characteristic of physiological sleep is not accompanied by a corresponding subsidence of sensorial memories, there results a veritable anarchy of ideas, because all control by the affectivities has ceased ; and we find that it is just because of this extreme incoherence and want of logic, so widely different from the mental characteristics of the same individual when awake, that dreams have always aroused the keen interest of psychologists, and constituted a problem which until now had resisted all attempts at its solution.

We may now briefly consider the advantages and

disadvantages of reasoning, as compared with those of actual experiment.

First of all we can easily see why, when reasoning starts from premises which are facts, it ought to lead to results also in accordance with facts. For if reasoning is nothing but a series of experiments, all of which, at least in theory, are capable of being performed, but which to save time and labour we merely imagine, it follows that *the logical process is only reality itself, brought into action by the imagination instead of in actual fact.* Therefore, it ceases to be a valid problem of philosophy to enquire " how it is possible that the logical process should give a valid representation of reality."

The problem would be a real one, if, after having been in contact with reality in its premises, reason should soar above it, and outside it, only to touch it again at the conclusion. But valid reasoning, far from losing contact with reality for an instant, *rests upon the solid ground of reality during all the phases of its development.*

As regards its advantages, one is very evident, namely, the enormous economy of time and labour effected by merely imagining the experiments, instead of actually carrying them out. Moreover, if the innumerable experiments which reason can perform in the imagination are in theory as possible as the similar experiments actually performed in the past, they are not always capable of being executed in practice. Reasoning can thus perform an infinitely larger number of experiments than would be possible if these experiments had to be really accomplished.

Further, in certain cases, reasoning has the advantage over actual experiment in yielding much more general results. If we ascertain by the use of a goniometer that the sum of the angles of a given triangle is equal to two right angles, we can deduce nothing as to the sum of the angles of other triangles, but by the series of the imagined experiments, which constitute the proof of this theorem, we are enabled to reach a result which is valid for all triangles.

This is, on the one hand, the consequence of the fact that the person who is reasoning is impelled, by the very nature of the psychic process which he is pursuing, to attribute to the results of his imagined experiments, as they take place in his mind, a more general validity than when he has really executed them in the past, for it is impossible to perform experiments in the imagination without attributing to them the results obtained from similar experiments in the past, which in this manner appear for the first time to be of broader validity, whilst there was no such necessity incumbent on the observer to give a general validity to the same result, when he has only verified it by actual experiment in one or two cases. This attribution of general validity to observed facts is the well-known process of *induction*, which is thus brought into action by the mere fact of reasoning.

On the other hand, when we perform imaginary experiments on a certain object, we can very rapidly perform a very large number of similar experiments, by varying in slight degree the conditions, so as to obtain an indefinite number of other objects belonging to the same category as the original object, but differing from it and from one another, and when thus we find that all these experiments lead to the same result, this latter acquires the broadest possible validity. A good instance of this is afforded when in imagination we vary in every possible way the inclination to two parallel lines of the line cutting them, and thus discover that in all cases alternate internal angles are equal to one another ; another instance of the same thing is when we alter in every possible way the shape of a triangle and find that the transference of the basal angles, so as to render them adjacent to the angle of the apex, is always possible and that the sum of the three angles is always equal to two right angles.

It is this possibility of compressing, so to speak, an infinite series of experiments into one experiment, which gives to the result, obtained by reasoning, a general validity, which the result of an experiment, which is actually performed, can never attain, because such an experiment can only be performed on one particular object.

Besides, the actual performance of experiments, where each experiment can be performed by itself, independently of all the others, involves the risk of presenting the various results of these experiments actually made as independent of one another, even when there is in reality a close connection between them.

Thus, the result of actually measuring the angles of a triangle with the goniometer, and finding that their sum is equal to two right angles, gives no information as to the dependence of this fact on the other fact, which is known as the postulate of Euclid. On the contrary, reasoning, which does not consist in the imagined performance of a single experiment (for this, if the experiment had actually been performed in the past, would tell us nothing new, and if it had not been performed we could not know its result beforehand), but the essence of which is a *new combination of past experiments*, succeeds in presenting final results as dependent on the results of these experiments in the past and so in demonstrating the bond which unites all these various facts with one another.

But though, in the aspects which we have just considered, reasoning is greatly superior to the actual carrying out of experiments, it is in other respects much inferior on account of the risks of error to which by its very nature it is exposed. Since at every step in the reasoning process it is necessary to generalise in the inductive manner the results of definite past experiments, there is always the danger of making an erroneous induction which would lead to a final result which would also be erroneous. At the same time, when the complexity of the combination of imagined experiments exceeds a certain limit, the person who reasons may not be able to follow in his imagination all the factors which come into play and their reciprocal effects, and therefore, by leaving some of them out of account, he may be led to an erroneous result.

Granted then these possible sources of error, and others also, which are examined in our work alluded to above, but which for want of time we cannot deal with here, we must admit that we can never have absolute confidence in the result of any combination of imagined experiments, especially if it is complex, and it is therefore always necessary, as John Stuart Mill so justly insists, to verify the results of reasoning, or at least some of them, by actual experiment.

It may appear at first sight that mathematical reasoning forms an exception to the rule that all reasoning is liable to error. But the greater relative certainty of mathematics is due to the fact that the objects with which it works have been, if not entirely constructed, at least greatly simplified by the very reason which employs them. They are thus endowed with definite, simple and well-known properties so that the risk of erroneous induction is reduced to a minimum. Further, the dangers resulting from the complexity of the combinations of imagined experiments are also diminished, on the one hand, by the simplicity characteristic of elementary mathematical reasoning, which results from the fact, that this reasoning has to do with the most simplified objects possible, and, on the other hand, because in advanced mathematical reasoning, the operator is safeguarded by the help afforded through the representation of each stage in the reasoning by suitable symbols. Then, too, one is rather apt to forget that certain mathematical reasonings, always the same, have been passed through the sieve of hundreds and hundreds of generations, and our confidence in their results is largely based on the infinitude of times that they have been controlled.

But, above all, we must not forget, as everyone knows who has made the smallest study of the history of mathematics, that many conclusions of mathematical reasoning, even due to the most eminent mathematicians, have been shown later to be erroneous, and thus it is clear that it is not true to say that mathematical reasoning is not liable to error.

There is another kind of inferiority which many have asserted to be peculiar to reasoning, as compared with actual experiment, and that is its *sterility*; but this kind of inferiority does not exist. It has been asserted that since reasoning must start from given premises consisting of known facts, and since the conclusion must be implicit in the premises, reasoning can therefore never produce new discoveries. Nothing could be more mistaken than this strange conclusion, especially when one recalls the masses of new facts discovered by pure reasoning alone, and above all in mathematics.

The error has arisen from the failure to perceive that the premises, which consist in the affirmation of facts which have been determined in the past, *do not at all imply the combination of these facts with one another in any given way*. Thus, in the case alluded to above, the known fact of the elongation of any given metallic rod under the influence of heat, and the other well ascertained fact that any given pendulum will oscillate more slowly than a shorter one, *do not in any way imply the operation or experiment of transporting a pendulum from a cold room to a warmer one*. This transportation has originated *a new historic succession of events*, freely created by my fancy, and this has led to the determination of a *new fact*, which can be really and properly termed a *new discovery*, namely, that a pendulum brought from a cold room into a warm one will oscillate more slowly. This is, we repeat, the determination of a new fact, which is in no way implicit in the premises alone, because to determine it, it is necessary to perform in imagination the experiment of a transportation, *and there is no indication of such an experiment in the premises.*

So the explanation of how it comes about that reasoning in general, and mathematical reasoning in particular, if the conclusion is really implicit in the premises, is not reducible to a pure and simple tautology (a question which Poincaré propounded to himself and which that great mathematician did not succeed in answering) is to be sought in the *creative act* of our imagination, which, under the stimulus of the corresponding affective tendency, calls into being new histories of things and new combinations of experiments, which, precisely because they are not contained in the premises, lead to the demonstration or discovery of really new facts.

Reasoning, therefore, in so far as it is a chain of imagined experiments combined with one another in the most various ways, can and does lead to discoveries, exactly as does a series of experiments actually carried out. Indeed, for reasons which we have examined in detail in our work already cited, but which we cannot indicate here, it proves to be much more fertile and productive than actual experiment.

We must now pass to the consideration of the higher forms of reasoning in order to show that the fundamental nature of all reasoning, which we have just sketched, remains unchanged also in them, and this we shall do in the next chapter.

CHAPTER XIII

BIOLOGICAL MEMORY AND THE FUNCTIONING OF THE
INTELLIGENCE (*Continued*)

Abstract reasoning. The ever wider application of the deductive method to science. Mathematical reasoning. The danger of mathematical mysticism which is showing itself in the fourth period of the evolution of mathematics characterised by symbolic inversion. Einstein's theory of relativity. The Syllogism. Mathematical Logic. Dialectical reasoning. Metaphysical reasoning. The different forms of our mentality. The single mnemonic property of living substance suffices to explain the whole of the operations of our intelligence.

AFTER having in the preceding chapter discussed the nature of reasoning in general, it remains for us to review the different higher forms of it, to which its continued evolution has given rise, and first of all we shall proceed to examine abstract reasoning.

ABSTRACT REASONING.

The operation of the affective tendencies, which, as we have seen, plays such a large part in the formation and determination of psychic phenomena, is just as clearly visible in the so-called process of abstraction.

Indeed, it would be easy to show that every abstract concept, from simple common nouns to the highest abstractions of science, is nothing but an " affective classification " of various objects, sensorially as

BIOLOGICAL MEMORY AND INTELLIGENCE

different from one another as one can imagine, but equivalent to one another with regard to a given affectivity, a definite utilitarian aim, or a given result which is either desired or feared. It follows that reasoning based on an abstract concept is equivalent by itself to all the concrete reasonings based on each of the objects or phenomena comprised in the abstract concept, and which in the absence of this concept it would be necessary to make.

These phenomena or objects having thus been shorn of all their attributes except the one which renders them equivalent from a given affective, utilitarian or scientific point of view, the corresponding concept is then represented by a single phenomenon or schematised object which is just what changes concrete into abstract reasoning. But the imagined operations or experiments with this object or phenomenon, thus schematised, continue to appear to the mind as " materially tangible " just as much as those of the concrete reasoning.

The formation of new concepts, which implies the discovery of new categories of objects equivalent to one another as regards the results of definite operations, leads thus to an increase in the number of experiments of which the results are known beforehand, and, in consequence of this knowledge, to an increase of the number of experiments which can be performed entirely in the imagination. At the same time, the schematisation of phenomena or objects, by making the experiments upon them much more simple, renders easier the mental representation of the long series of these experiments, connected as they are with one another in the most varied ways. As a consequence, for these two reasons, the final result of the passage from concrete to abstract reasoning is the ever wider application of the deductive method in science.

But in proportion as the series of imagined experiments becomes longer and more complicated, so the difficulty of following them is increased, if every process has to be performed mentally without being supported by any visible representation. From this difficulty there arises the necessity of inventing and using *graphic symbols* which grow ever more complicated, in order to keep before the mind the results of the various experiments which have to be performed in the imagination. These symbols keep in some sense bodily in view those results which have been obtained by previous mental combinations and which constitute points of departure for further combinations ; and so they aid the imagination in grasping and envisaging with a single glance all the inter-connected chain of these combinations, including even the most complex of them ; *in a word, they serve as a schematic tangible representation on which the mental process as it proceeds can project itself.*

All this symbolism has thus been made necessary by the increasing complexity and wider application of the deductive method in the so-called exact sciences, and it, too, has become more and more complicated till it has often hidden the true and essential nature of reasoning ; this nature, which consists in being a chain of simple imagined experiments, has nevertheless remained unchanged under the veil of obscurity with which it has been enveloped by symbolism.

MATHEMATICAL REASONING.

This, then, is what we have striven to prove in the chapters of our work cited above, which are devoted to mathematical reasoning, but which we cannot find space to repeat here even in brief summary. We shall only mention the four principal stages into which we have thought it possible to divide this, the highest form of reasoning.

The first stage, viz., that of *direct symbolism*, is that anterior to the introduction of positive and negative numbers, and in consequence of the direct correspondence between the symbol and the reality which it represents, it is in this stage that the true nature of the reasoning process as described above is most clearly displayed. The next stage, that of *indirect symbolism*, after the introduction of positive and negative numbers, since in certain cases it gives rise to " imaginary numbers," seems at first sight to contradict the general nature of reasoning considered as a series of imagined tangible experiments, but this contradiction vanishes when we notice that the imaginary and complex numbers are nothing but the analytic representatives of *direction*, and that they also consequently possess a meaning which is empirically tangible not less than the so-called " real " numbers.

The third stage, viz., that of *symbolic condensation*, begins with the infinitesimal calculus, and it is specially characterised by the fact that, whilst in elementary algebra every operation has its representative symbol, in the calculus different series of operations, each of which may even be made up of an infinite series of operations succeeding one another in a given determinate order, are represented by one condensed symbol. The difficulties in the comprehension and use of mathematics which had already increased in the passage from the first to the second stage, are still more augmented as we pass to the third stage. This is due to the fact that symbolic condensation, even more than indirect symbolism, tends to make the contact between the symbol and the reality which it represents more indirect, to render their mutual relations more complicated and to remove thus the solid support given to the person reasoning, when he can see clearly at every moment behind the symbol the tangible empirical operations which this represents, and which here as before constitute the essence of the reasoning process.

The fourth stage, finally, is what we have termed the stage of *symbolic inversion* ; it is particularly interesting because by introducing and developing the custom (very useful in certain cases) of giving geometrical names by way of analogy to purely algebraic expressions to which there is no corresponding geometrical reality, in a word, by creating a geometry of four or more dimensions, it has given rise to a veritable mathematical metaphysic or mysticism. Forgetful of the ends which this symbolic inversion has been invented to serve, certain mathematicians have attempted to give a geometrical or physical meaning, of which our intelligence is unable to form the dimmest conception, to certain algebraic expressions which by symbolic inversion have received geometrical and physical names. This mathematical metaphysic has received a new lease of life by the appearance of Einstein's theory of relativity, in which Einstein speaks, as if they really corresponded to something real, of a four-dimensional " space," in which the fourth dimension is time, of the " curvature " of our three dimensional space, of " tensors " of this four dimensional space and so on.

So long as the relativists persist in materialising such shadows and in affirming the physical reality of their purely algebraic entities, which in the eyes of these mystics become mysterious transcendental substances, they will be certainly not justified in boasting that they have succeeded in " explaining " the phenomena for which the theory itself has been constructed. " Explaining," in the psychological sense, means obtaining certain facts by the mental combination of other simpler and more familiar facts. Now, if in order to explain certain physical or astronomical phenomena, we have recourse to a " space " of four dimensions, to a " curvature " of our space and to other similar conceptions, which not only are not familiar to us, but which our mind, formed as it has been by our Euclidean three-dimensional space, is unable to picture even in the most distant way, this is certainly not to give an explanation at all. The theory of relativity, so far, has remained a purely mathematical construction.

corresponding to which there must be some physical reality seeing that some of its results seem to have been confirmed by experiment or observation. But the task of the relativists now is to seek to discover in what this physical reality consists, so as to render it capable of being grasped by our imagination. It is only when they have succeeded in doing this that they will have the right to claim that they have really " explained " the facts, for the explanation of which their theory was invented.

SYLLOGISM AND MATHEMATICAL LOGIC.

We have already seen that reasoning, in so far as it is a connected series of imagined experiments, necessarily involves for each of these a process of induction, by means of which the results, obtained by certain experiments actually carried out in the past, are generalised so as to be applicable to the similar particular experiment which at the moment is being imagined. Once this combining of imagined experiments has been accomplished by the constructive fancy, and we have thus been enabled to follow the various vicissitudes of the object in which we are interested, our attention, which has hitherto been concentrated on the creative act of reasoning, may be directed to the path followed by this reasoning, in order to control and verify by the careful recall of personal memories, whether at every step in the process the result attributed to each experiment is really correct, that is, whether each of the inductions on which the reasoning is based is legitimate. Thus we obtain a different mode of distribution of the attention, which serves to render explicit each of these inductions, that is, to bring each of them in turn into strong relief *as the premise of a syllogism*, which is nothing but the assigning of a given object to a certain class, or the inclusion of a whole class of objects witnin another class. The mental procedure is briefly as follows : this or that object, or all the objects of this or that class, having been submitted to a given experiment, are found to possess the characteristics of this or that other class.

It follows that reasoning assumes in this phase the syllogistic form, which consists of definite classificatory operations, such as inclusions, reunions, and intersections of classes, performed on materials produced and presented to the mind by the precedent creative acts due to the constructive fancy. This form of deduction based on operations with classes, into which any kind of reasoning may be transformed, is nothing but the formation of a kind of catalogue of the results of definite experiments, after these have been mentally executed by the creative imagination. It resembles the anatomical dissection of an organ after the function of the organ has built up its complicated structure. In other words, it is a *static* method of considering the results of a *dynamic* process.

The fact that, owing to the induction which lies at the base of all reasoning, it is possible to dissect any given piece of reasoning into operations of inclusions or reunions or intersections of classes, allows us to regard these operations as experiments of a general kind applicable to all kinds of reasoning. At the same time, they are classificatory operations familiar to every day experience, such as that of the " contained content," of which we all know the results beforehand, and which consequently may at once be carried out mentally.

These mental operations of inclusions, reunions and intersections of classes consequently give rise to results of a general character, valid for all kinds of reasoning considered in their static aspect. To this extent, they embody " the fundamental principles of reasoning " and constitute " pure logic "; in other words, they are a universal mode of reasoning applicable to all possible cases, which constitute merely so many particular applications of these principles. Language with its propositions and syllogistic processes on the one hand, and mathematical logic with its symbols and its algebraical transformations on the other hand, each striving to express adequately these operations on classes, constitute together " formal logic," that is to say, the form which clothes pure logic in words or in algebraical symbols.

Great were the hopes to which this investiture of the old classical logic with a form similar to that of mathematics gave rise in the first phases of its development ; for the resemblance of external forms raised the hope that the productivity of the new mathematical logic would equal or surpass the marvellous productivity of the mathematical calculus.

But disappointment was not long in coming ; it could not be otherwise, as we have easily demonstrated in our work cited above. For if mathematical logic, in so far as it aimed at becoming a system of steno-ideographic transcription for international comprehension, to be used especially in mathematical treatises, as it was by Prof. Peano and some few other mathematicians, seems to have attained the end for which it was introduced (an end of which it is easy to exaggerate the importance, considering the few individuals who make use of it), and if it may sometimes be of use as a rigorous control of logical reasoning, it was easy on the other hand for us to demonstrate that since it gives no support to the creative imagination, it is condemned by its very nature to complete sterility as a method of discovery of fresh truth ; and we insisted that it is consequently psychologically quite erroneous to expect from logical symbolism, even in small degree, the immense advantages which the introduction of symbolism has conferred on mathematics.

INTENTIONAL REASONING : DIALECTIC AND
METAPHYSICS.

Whilst in the forms of reasoning previously examined, which we may term productive or constructive, the object of the person reasoning is either to predict by a suitable series of imagined experiments, that is by means of certain histories of things fashioned by his constructive imagination, the results which will follow from some of his actions, or, in a more general way, to discover hitherto unknown truths, that is new derivations of one set of phenomena from another, in " intentional reasoning," on the other

229

hand, the person reasoning does not seek to discover what the truth is, but strives to demonstrate the validity of definite affirmations which he is much concerned to uphold.

Moreover, when the reasoning individual fashions by his creative fancy new combinations of imagined experiments, as he does in the forms of reasoning which we have previously examined, he constructs thus new histories of things and discovers—if only mentally—real new facts, which enrich the stores of human knowledge, just as much as does the researcher in the laboratory with the experiments which he actually carries out. But when a person reasons "intentionally," he seeks less to discover new facts than to classify or present well-known phenomena in one manner rather than in another.

It is easy to demonstrate the classificatory character of dialectical reasoning, one of the two fundamental varieties of " intentional reasoning," especially if we choose for our example the dialectic of the bar, in which all the efforts of the person reasoning are directed towards placing a given individual or a given fact in one rather than in another of the pigeon-holes of that great distributing bureau of human and social facts constituted by the civil and penal codes of law.

It follows that, whereas in constructive reasoning the syllogism has only the secondary function of controlling the legitimacy of the various inductions on which the reasoning is being built up, in dialectical reasoning, on the contrary, the syllogism takes on a part of primary importance, namely, to direct the attention of the hearer or reader solely to those attributes of the object or phenomenon under consideration which render it capable of being placed in the class in which the person reasoning desires to put it. In other words, the syllogism appears to have the purpose of leading the hearer or reader to form one "mental perception" of the object rather than another—or, better expressed, to lead him to complete his mental perception of it in the direction which particularly interests the person who is reasoning, since this "mental perception" so completed will lead to the desired classification of the object in question.

The aim of the primary affective tendency becomes in this case to recall, select and maintain before the mind only those atrtibutes of the phenomenon or object which complete the desired "mental perception," whilst the function of the secondary affective tendency is now no longer to recall, select, and emphasise other attributes contrary to those which are desired, as it does in the case of constructive reasoning, but rather to watch, less any attribute might be overlooked which might help in the desired classification, and that no attribute inconsistent with the desired thesis might be accidentally recalled.

In intentional reasoning two antagonistic classifications or presentations, upheld respectively by two opposing dialecticians, have each its definite end to serve. It follows that in the majority of disputes of this character it is by no means necessary that one or the other of two contradictory affirmations should be true and the other false, as is the case in constructive reasoning where a given combination can only lead to one definite result. Since the two opposed statements are really two "directed" revivals of memories, two different "choices," it entirely depends on the end sought for, which is to be preferred to the other.

Thus there is an essential psychological difference between constructive and dialectical reasoning. But it is just the identity of the syllogistic investment with which both are clothed (one in an accessory, the other in a necessary way), which has hitherto prevented psychologists from discovering and emphasising this essential difference.

Metaphysical reasoning, which is the other form of "intentional" reasoning, seeks, like dialectical reasoning, to attain an end and pursues it by analogous methods. Metaphysical reasoning is thus also a process of intentional presentation, but instead of dealing, like dialectical reasoning, with definite phenomena, it seeks to attain a comprehensive view of the entire universe (Weltanschauung) which shall conform to the deepest desires of the human mind. The ardent and irresistible desire to represent the world to himself and to others not as it is, but as he would like it to be, is what drives the metaphysician to transcend reality, to place himself outside it, and even to deny it in order to construct and uphold his system.

Consequently, differing in this respect profoundly from the positivist, he feels the necessity of penetrating into the "essential nature" of phenomena, in order to discover or to create the illusion of discovering some intelligent and purposeful cause of these phenomena on which he would like to see reality based. He is unable to discover, either in immediate experience or in the " material " representation of reality provided by science, any satisfaction for his particular aspirations, and regarding not unjustly scientific experiments and theories as so many disproofs of what he would fain see existing, he exerts all his strength to transcend the empirical barriers which block the passage to his aspirations, and he harbours the illusion that reason and reasoning can succeed in this task by the use of " transcendental concepts." All, however, that he succeeds in doing, as we have tried to show in our work cited above, is to borrow concepts from reality and then to empty them of the greater part of their content so as to make them amenable to the greatest possible elasticity of interpretation, in order to avoid their too obvious collisions with reality.

These concepts thus deprived of any relation to real phenomena, these ideas thus dematerialised which, just for that reason, eventually become totally unintelligible, serve to provide the metaphysician with the illusion that he has transcended experience and has discovered outside it that condition of the universe which his soul longs for.

There is no other form of reasoning in which the primary importance of the affective tendencies in their function of guiding and modelling the operations of reason appears with greater clarity than in metaphysics.

Conclusion.

The Functioning of Intelligence in Relation to the Purposefulness of Life

It remains for us to examine how all the different forms of our mentality are due to the affective tendencies, how for instance positivists and meta-physicians, synthetic and analytic, intuitive and logical, classical and romantic minds, all owe their different intellectual qualities to the affective peculiar-ities of their psyche. But here again we must refer to our work mentioned above, in order to pass on to draw the general conclusion from all that has gone before.

This conclusion is as follows :

The operations of our intelligence are entirely made up of the reciprocal actions of two primary fundamental activities of our psyché, viz., sensory activities and affective activities. The first consist in sensations and the simple mnemonic recall of sensations, the second in the aspirations or strivings of our minds towards definite ends. It follows that those faculties which have hitherto been con-sidered by the majority of philosophers to be of a purely intellectual character, such as attention, imagination, classification, abstraction, reasoning, coherence, logicality, criticism, and so on, appear to us to be at bottom of an affective nature.

Affective activity seems, therefore, to us to mingle itself with all the manifestations of our thought. One might even term this affective activity the sole constructive power of our mind, which, using as materials the simple memories stored in our sensory mnemonic accumulations, erects all the edifices of reason from that of the lowest animal to that of the man of lofty genius.

But this affective faculty which thus reveals itself to us as at once the mighty builder, awakener, guide and moderator of our intelligence, is in its turn a manifestation of the mnemonic property which is the fundamental characteristic of all living substance ; nay, more, it is its most characteristic and direct manifestation.

Consequently, the mnemonic faculty which has appeared to us as yielding an explanation of the most fundamental biological phenomena which exhibit purposefulness : from the predetermined morpho-logical adaptation of organisms, from ontogenetic development which constructs organs which can only fulfil their function in a future adult state, from the inheritability of acquired characters of which ontogenetic development and phylogenetic evolution are the results, down to the most simple and most " mechanised " reflexes so well preadapted to the preservation of the individual, and to the most complex instincts in virtue of which animals provide for future environmental conditions of which they know nothing, this same faculty now reveals itself as the explanation of all the most varied manifesta-tions of our psychic life as well.

As Archimedes required only a fulcrum for his lever in order to move the world, so the mnemonic property—which at bottom is nothing more than the power of reproducing by internal causes the same physiological states as were at first produced by the forces of the external world—is alone sufficient to enable vital energy to give rise to all the characteristic purposeful manifestations of life, including the whole thinking and reasoning apparatus of the soul.

It is, therefore, exclusively this mnemonic property which gives to life its purposeful aspect which differentiates it essentially from every phenomenon of the inorganic world, since it alone is moved, not only by forces " *a tergo*," but also by forces " *a fronte.*"

The aim which man, moved by his affective tendencies, strives to attain, the environment which the animal prepares to meet by the complex behaviour of its instinct, the environmental conditions to which the organ of the embryo formed in the maternal womb will become adapted, act now as " pulls from in front " (*vis a fronte*) because they acted as " *vis a tergo* " in the past, since the physiological activities then evoked in the organism by these external circumstances, have left behind them, as traces of themselves, mnemonic accumulations, which now are what constitute the real and effective " *vis a tergo*," which directs and actuates the development, the instinct, and the whole conscious conduct of the living being.

And all the operations of intelligence put in action by one or other of the primary affective tendencies, continually controlled by the secondary affective tendency of the corresponding state of attention, impelled by the interest in definite objects to perform on them a series of imagined experiments, and then guided, still by affectivities, to pass from the most rudimentary intuitive and concrete forms of reasoning to the most elevated and abstract varieties of scientific deduction, sometimes held to the solid ground of the real by watchful prudence, and sometimes driven by deep and irresistible feeling to the most nebulous metaphysical speculation, all these varied, complex and proteiform functions of the intelligence are at once the highest and the most characteristic manifestations of the purposeful aspect of life.

CHAPTER XIV

Conclusion : The Biological Memory and the Moral Problem

The mnemonic conception of life is the only one which provides us with a comprehensive view of all biological and psychic phenomena. On account of this mnemonic property the evolution of life is not a simple transformation, but a continuous progress. With the progressive complication of the affective tendencies and with the growth of social life, which goes hand in hand with the development of the intelligence, there arises in man the moral question, both individual and social. This question resolves itself into the other question, how to attain the greatest possible harmony of life ? Owing to the mnemonic property, biological and social, our moral efforts will persist as active factors in the future even long after our own ephemeral existences have terminated. To each one, we may say, there is thus granted an intensity and duration of the survival of his soul, proportionate to the altruistic result obtained by his own efforts. The positivist finds in his own nature, in the thrilling surge and joyful display of all life, the supreme reason for his conduct and the deepest satisfaction of his own conscience.

THE conception of life as a peculiar form of energy endowed in contradistinction to all other forms of energy with the property of mnemonic accumulation, which has permitted us to extend the mnemonic theory which was at first applied only to ontogenetic development, to all the purposeful manifestations of life, including instincts, affective tendencies, and even thought in its most complex form, is the only one which enables us to take a comprehensive view of all biological and psychical phenomena, which we consequently consider to be of the same fundamental nature, but which are sharply distinguished from those which belong to the physico-chemical world.

In the midst of the age-long strife between vitalistico-animistic theories and physico-chemical theories, each vainly seeking from opposite standpoints to explain the enigma of life, the mnemonic theory represents a middle point of view which we may term vitalistico-energetic, which takes into consideration and endeavours to reconcile the contradictory assertions of these two opposite theories of life.

At the same time, the hypothesis of mnemonic accumulation, aided by the supplementary hypothesis of a " centro-epigenesis," that is, of a " formative radiation from a centre," allows us to catch a glimpse of the mechanism of the inheritance of acquired characters, and thus deprives the struggle for existence and natural selection of their appearance of being the sole and inevitable means by which organic evolution can continue to progress.

According to this mnemonic theory, the incessant efforts of living beings to adapt themselves ever better to external conditions no longer appears as a vain labour of Sisyphus, which must be begun anew by every fresh generation ; but, on the contrary, we become convinced that every victory of life, every success obtained in its effort to make and maintain a place for itself, and to expand amongst the other forms of energy of the physico-chemical cosmos, far from being lost, becomes converted into a permanent gain.

Consequently, whilst in the evolution of the inorganic world, we find only a simple *transformation* of one mode of being into another which is only substituted for the preceding one, so that no past condition persists as an active agent in the future, the evolution of the organic world, on the contrary, is a continual *progress*. This progress consists in more and more perfect adaptation, and therefore in a progressively greater expansion and intensification of this latest " intruder " which is life, into the general energetic system of the universe.

Thus, in the evolution of species, we encounter a continually greater complication and perfection of morphological structure, ever better fitted to triumph over the adverse contingencies of the external world, and in the complex instincts of animals we contemplate with admiration the different progressive varieties of behaviour stereotyped in their finest details, by means of which animals ever better provide in advance for future conditions of the environment of which they know nothing.

So, in man, we behold a morphological structure which, viewed in its entirety, is the most complicated and perfect in the whole organic world, and which includes the brain, an organ of intelligence of ever-increasing size. The importance of this organ and of its function, the intelligence, is so great that it nearly succeeds in reversing the conditions of adaptation of life to the environment. For whereas in animals adaptation is purely passive, in the sense that the animal becomes changed in accordance with the environment, in man adaptation becomes an active process, in the sense that man, by the aid of science and technical skill, adapts the environment to himself. It is perhaps not yet possible fully to forsee the future consequences of this reversal of the process of adaptation in their influence on the greater expansion and intensification of life.

This enormous development of the intelligence, which has succeeded in opening an impassable chasm between man and other animals, implies, as we have already seen, as antecedent or concomitant or subsequent phenomena, the most varied complications of the affective tendencies, in which the vital activity manifests itself in the most intense manner. At the same time, it impels man to develop his social life and to extend and intensify his relations with his fellows. Thus is brought into being, for the first time with the appearance of man, the *ethical conception*, both in its individual and social aspects.

Now, if we enquire in what, in its final analysis, the essence and progress of *individual* morality consists, as it is customarily preached and understood, we find that its aim is nothing more than the harmonious development and satisfaction of the affective substratum of our psyche, and it is likewise in the harmonious development and satisfaction of the various personal desires and individual interests of all the members of the community that the progress of *social* morality consists.

There still remains, indeed, much disharmony and reciprocal inhibition between many of our affective tendencies ; the contest of our inner passions is often tragic ; there is usually a conflict between the desire for immediate pleasure, especially for excessive pleasure of the sensual kind, and the desire to escape future ills and pains both physical and moral ; there is also a conflict between the feverish pursuit of present material blessings and the longing for spiritual benefits which can only be attained in the future. Now, individual morality progresses in proportion as it can replace these conflicts by the greatest possible harmony of our affective nature, and this affective harmony can only be attained by education and manifests itself in the peace and happiness of the individual.

In the same way, we find want of harmony and antagonism between the interests of the various individuals or groups of individuals who contend with one another within the bosom of the society. The egoistic interest of the individual is often opposed to the collective interests. Capitalist exploitation of the working class has produced the misery, suffering and brutalisation of a large part of that class, and in consequence has given rise to class-conflict which can easily degenerate into class hatred ; and the conflict of national interests has let loose that curse of humanity, fratricidal war between the nations. Now social morality, in so far as it is embodied in the supreme principles of equity—whether these be expressed by the Ten Commandments, the Gospel precepts, or the categorical imperative of Kant— progresses in proportion as it succeeds in replacing these conflicts by the greatest possible harmony of individual interests, both with those of other in- dividuals and with those of the community, and thus in promoting the greatest happiness of the greatest number of our fellows.

We thus see that the principles of individual morality and those of social justice are directed towards assisting the fundamental tendency of life towards its own preservation and expansion, and that in the final analysis they may be summarised in the lessening of suffering, which is suspension, arrest, or cessation of life. In every act of benevolence or of justice, which strives to replace with concord a conflict which was the cause of suffering, we obey this fundamental biological tendency, and we identify ourselves with all living beings. We no longer live our egoistic and mean individual lives, but we palpitate in unison with the quivering joy of all life.

Let us strive then to mingle our own lives and those of our children and our other dearest kinsmen with the great river of all life, without stopping the least portion of it in order to make room for ourselves. Do not let us seek our happiness at the expense of that of others, but let us work so that our weal shall be all addition and profit to the common stock, without anything to be taken away or added on the debit side. Let us pride ourselves not in being sufficient only for ourselves, but in contributing to the utmost extent of our ability to the increase of the well-being and happiness of others.

Do not let us descend to our particular acts of benevolence or of justice by starting from too abstract a categorical imperative, the justification of which we may perhaps search for in vain, but let us, on the contrary, rise step by step towards the ideal of this imperative, beginning with humble acts of goodness or elementary deeds of justice, the reason for which it never occurs to us to ask ourselves, because in the relief of our neighbour's suffering and in the new joy which we have afforded him, we feel the pulse of our own lives accelerated and strengthened.

Do not let this goal seem to us too modest, for, alas! unlimited is the amount of human suffering still to be assuaged, numberless are the social conflicts still to be reconciled, and long is the path still to be traversed and hard are the battles to be fought before we succeed in establishing a system of true social justice and of complete peace between all nations.

Do not let us be discouraged by the apparent vanity of our efforts or by the brevity of our lives. The mnemonic property of the biological organism, which is reflected and reinforced in the social organism, brings it about that every scientific or technical discovery which constitutes an advance in the adaptation of life to any given environment, every act of goodness or of justice which replaces a vital conflict with a new vital harmony, every new creation of the artist which excites feelings of sweetness and love even in hostile minds, far from being lost with the death of its author, persists as an active agent in the future, far beyond our ephemeral material existence. The discoveries of Volta and Watt, of Jenner and Pasteur, still help to augment human happiness and diminish suffering; the word of Christ is still heard, loftily severe or infinitely sweet, as a demand for justice or as a plea for peace amongst men who rend each other for mere material interests. A melody of Bellini still awakens in a thousand souls the same sweet emotion, which delighted Bellini himself in the moment of his sublime inspiration. That which constituted the real and exquisite essence of the minds and hearts of these great men survives still and preserves its character intact, even though centuries have elapsed since their bodies crumbled to dust.

But even more humble lives, whether they are devoted to the production of new material means of existence and comfort, adapted to make the environment more favourable to the preservation, expansion and elevation of human life, or whether they are engaged in the propagation of scientific, technical, hygienic or economic truths constituting more perfect adaptations of man to his environment ; even any act of goodness, however humble and unnoticed, which succeeds in awakening in some soul the enduring sweetness of a feeling of gratitude, even the most simple act of justice which succeeds in permanently extinguishing a desire for vengeance or a feeling of hate, even the most modest musical performance which has caused a note of tenderness or of aspiration towards the ideal to pulsate amidst rough surroundings still far from being elevated—none of these humble deeds, which are well within the powers of the most modest individual, are never totally lost, since the mnemonic property of the biological and social life preserves them and adds them one to another and sends them forth to echo, ever dispensing good, to the most distant centuries.

Each one of us, as we may so express it, can thus acquire for what constitutes the very essence of his soul an intensity and duration of survival, proportionate to the altruistic result which his efforts have achieved, and, in the same way, each one can aid in prolonging the spiritual existence of his dear dead ones, and in feeling them live again in him, in proportion as his actions and feelings are inspired by those of their feelings and acts which are the most beneficial for future generations.

Therefore, whilst the metaphysician and the believer feel the need—which we must all respect—of seeking the support and inspiration of their conduct in some Being, outside themselves and immensely greater than they, Who knows and wills, Who, as they think, pursues His own eternal purpose and directs the whole universe towards this end, the positivist, who does not subject reason to feeling and who cannot accept by an act of faith that which his reason shows him to be false and even absurd, is able to look serenely in the face of reality as it actually appears to him. In vain the positivist has searched the inanimate world : he has been totally unable to discover in it any signs of purpose ; but he does not rebel against this discovery, as do the metaphysician and the believer, rather he accepts it with resignation, the more readily, as he finds in his own nature, and even more securely, the supreme reason for his conduct and the very support of his life. He discovers it—indeed he feels it—in the joyous quivering of all life, a minute but vigorous pulse of which is in himself, in his flesh and blood, and in his mind and soul.

THE MORAL PROBLEM

In submitting to the inexorable laws of his own nature, in harmonising his life with all life, in possessing the consciousness of having done all that was humanly possible to increase the opportunities for life in general, to diminish the sufferings and pains of his fellows, and to cause a little more justice and love to prevail amongst men, he succeeds in finding in the response made to him by the inner voice of his conscience the deepest and sweetest satisfaction, and he becomes persuaded that not in vain has been lighted for him, even if only for a brief instant, the torch of life.

INDEX

Abstraction, 234.
Abstract reasoning, 220 ff.
Accumulators, 51, 70, 82, 5, 98, 105.
Accumulation, specific, 85, 90, 91 ff., 100 ff., 119, 153.
Acquired characters, inheritance of, 27, 119; non-transmissibility of, 31; inheritability of, 33.
Adaptation, 176; phenomena of, 151; morphological, 172, 235.
Affection, family, 161, 205.
Affective impulses, 142; tendencies, 142 and *passim*.
Affective transference, 205; classification, 220; harmony, 242.
Affectivities, 158, 165, 193, 208, 212, 221, 234.
Algebra, 224.
Altruism, 166.
Animism, 134.
Appetites, 148, 176.
Archimedes, 235.
Arms, 164.
Artist, 244.
Assimilation, 35, 103 f.
Association of ideas, 101; limitation of, 101.
Atavism, 48 f., 75.
Attention, 206 ff., 227, 234.
Autonomy, ontogenetic, 75.
Attraction, sexual, 158.
Auto-plasmation, 132 f.

Bain, 163, 165.
Baldwin, 169.
Beauty, 174.
Behaviour, 142, 149.
Bellini, 245.
Benevolence, 234 f.
Bernard, Claude, 92, 94, 106.
Biochemists, 197.

Biogen hypothesis, 97.
Biogenesis, 34, 74, 79, 82, 90.
Biological organism, 244; life, 245; phenomena, 238.
Biology, 35, 83.
Birds, nestbuilding of, 114, 117.
Blastomeres, 40 f., 44, 46, 54 ff., 58, 62.
Blood, 181; circulation of, 29, 78.
Born, 44, 46.
Bottazzi, Filippo, 176, 187 f., 192, 194, 195 f., 199.
Brailsford, 179.
Braus, 75, 77.
Butler, 34, 79.

Capacity factor, 95, 99.
Calculus, 224; infinitesimal, 223.
Caterpillars, pupation of, 113.
Causes, 188 ff.
Cellular specialization, 35; proliferation, 67.
Cerebral cortex, 155.
Central zone of development, 45 f., 59, 69, 71 f., 73 f., 76.
Centro-epigenesis, 45 f., 60, 68, 72, 75 ff., 119, 123.
Chabry, 54.
Charging current, 153.
Christ, 244.
Chemical energy, 136 f.
Ciamician, 98.
Class conflict, 242; hatred, 242.
Classification, 234; affective 220.
Claypole, 112.
Colloidal system, 179, 190.
Compensatory growth, 66.
Composition, 166.
Comte, 190.
Concepts, 221; Transcendental, 233.
Concrete reasoning, 221 f.

249   R

INDEX

INDEX

Nägeli, 32, 122.
Natural philosophers, 107 f., selection, 26, 28, 31 ff.
Neo-Darwinism, 26, 31, 73.
Neo-Lamarckism, 26, 73.
Nervous circulation, 124 ; current, 74, 81, 86, 88 ff., 93, 153 ; energy, 51, 62, 64 ff. ; transmission of, 128 ; impulses, 127 ; shocks, 96, 98 ; system, 77, 128, 150, 155.
Nervomotive force, 98 f., 106.
Neurones, 95, 100, 102.
Non-representative material, 47.
Nostalgia, 156, 160, 205.
Nuclear division, 39, 53, 57 f., 62 f. ; energy, 64 ; specialisation, 39, 53, 56 ff. ; stimulation, 61, 64, 76.
Numbers, 223.
Nurselings, 157.
Nutrition, 70 f.

Ontogeny, 33 f., 43, 52, 67 f., 74, 79 f., 82, 86, 116, 172, 187, 238.
Ontology, 198.
Organic world, 177 ; system, 195.
Origin of species, 122, 126.
Orr, 34, 79.
Orthogenetic theories, 32.
Ostriches, newly-hatched, 112.
Ostwald, 88, 107, 142.

Pananimism, 129.
Pangenes, 23, 123.
Paranoiacs, 211.
Parasitism, 204.
Particulate inheritance, 28, 48 f.
Parturition, 157.
Pasteur, 244.
Pauly, 130, 132, 134 f.
Peano, Prof., 229.
Peasants 164.
Perception, mental, 231.
Pfeffer, 60 ff., 65.
Phlegmatics, 99.
Phylogeny, 33, 74, 79, 82, 89 f., 124, 131.
Physical energy, 94, 131.
Physico-chemical energy, 96, 108 ; laws, 173, 175 f., 187, 189, 194 ; phenomena, 93 f., 139, 154.

Physiological condition, 148 f., 169, 172, 176, 188 f., 193, 197, 204 ; equilibrium, 192 ff. ; invariability, 149 f. ; phenomena, 192, 199 f. ; stability, 191.
Piéron, 152.
Pillon, 159.
Plants 125 ff. 129, 189.
Plasmatic influence, 41, 45.
Plasmolysis, 60.
Pleasure, 242.
Poincaré, 218.
Polymorphism, 75.
Positivists, 234, 246.
Posthumous action, 76.
Potential elements, 85 ; specific, 86 f., 91 ; energy, 71, 93.
Pregnancy, 157.
Preformation, 38 ff., 43 ff., 47 ff., 75.
Protomeres, 81, 118.
Protista, 194.
Protoplasm, 180.
Psychiatry, 203.
Psychic acts, 139.
Psychic memory, 80 f., 92., 119, 154.
Psychology, 35, 101, 199 f., 203, 238.
Psychologist, 202, 206, 212, 232.
Purposefulness, 141 ff., 166 ff., 180, 184, 191, 198, 200 f., 204, 234, 237.

Quinton, 149.

Rana Esculanta, 44.
Reactivation, 152.
Reason, 173.
Reasoning, 209 ff., 220 f., 228, 233 f. ; abstract, 221 f. ; constructive, 232 ; dialectical, 232 ; mathematical, 217, 223 ; metaphysical, 232.
Reflexes, 170, 172, 191.
Regeneration, 40 ff., 56, 117.
Rejuvenation, 103, 106.
Rejuvenescence, 83.
Relativists, 225 f.
Relativity, 225.
Representative current, 89.
Reproduction, 103.
Reproductive cells, 78, 81.
Repulsive reaction, 143.

252

INDEX

Reserve idioplasm, 40, 42 f.
Respiratory system, 195, 198.
Ribbert, 67.
Ribot, 147, 159 f., 165, 193, 208, 212, 221, 234.
Rignano, 176 ff.
Robertson, 179,
Roux, Wilhelm, 33, 40, 44, 46, 67, 137.

Spectrum, 105.
Spencer, Herbert, 31, 48, 107, 160 f.
Spirit, 178.
Spiritualism, 199.
Spontaneous variation, 48.
Stability, 180.
Stationary state, 88.
Stirp, 29.
Structural adaptation, 32.
Suffering, 244, 247.
Survival, 246.
Syllogism, 227, 230 f.
Symbiosis, 156 f., 204.
Symbolism, 222 f., 229.
Symbols, 224, 228.
Symbolic condensation, 223 f. ; inversion, 224 f.
Synapse, 78.
Synthesis, biological, 201.
Synthetic views, 185.
Schiff, 143.
Schopenhauer, 147.
Schultze, Oscar, 55.
Science, 173.
Secretion, Glandular, 187 ; irritating, 157.
Seduction, 162.
Self-preservation, Instinct of, 148.
Semon, 80, 90, 109 ff.
Sensations, 93, 96, 144, 203, 206, 208, 234.
Sergi, 206
Sernon, 34.
Sensory memories, 205, 210, 212.
Schematisation, 221.
Sexual act, 147 ; attraction, 158 ; cells, 31 ; desires, 176 ; hunger, 162 ; instinct, 146 f., 200, 204.

Sherrington, 170, 206.
Sleep, 212.
Sociability, 161, 205.
Social justice, 243 f. ; progress, 174.
Soma, 29.
Somatic elements, 58 f., 86.
Soul, 178, 186, 246.
Specific accumulation, 173, 177 ; current, 93 ; energy, 92 ; potentiality, 51, 58, 91.

Teratology, 50.
Thirst, 144, 176, 204.
Thought, 238.
Transference, 162 ff., 205 ; Affective, 205.
Transcendentalism, 233.
Transformation of species, 25.
Transmissibility of acquired characters, 35, 82 ; of stimuli, 128.
Troglodytes, 150.
Trophic action, 83 ; nervous energy, 84 ; stimuli, 137.

Unicellular animals, 46, 63, 76.

Van Bemmelen, 179.
Variations, 32.
Vertebrates, 30, 46, 77.
Vinci, Leonardo da, 180.
Vis a fronte, 171 f. ; a tergo, 171 f.
Visceral sensation, 155, 177.
Vital conflict, 244 ; energy, 51, 70, 98, 104, 134, 136, 236 ; harmony, 244 ; phenomena, 35 ff., 80 f., 83, 90, 104, 130, 173, 180, 183, 197.
Vitalism, 135, 139 f.
Volta, 244.

Wallace, Alfred Russel, 122.
Wundt, 93.
War, 242.
Watt, 244.
Weismannian continuity, 32.
Whitman, 43.
Will, 133, 147, 206, 207 ; power, 99.
Zoja, Raffaele, 54